AF579887

# Patients
## AND METHODS

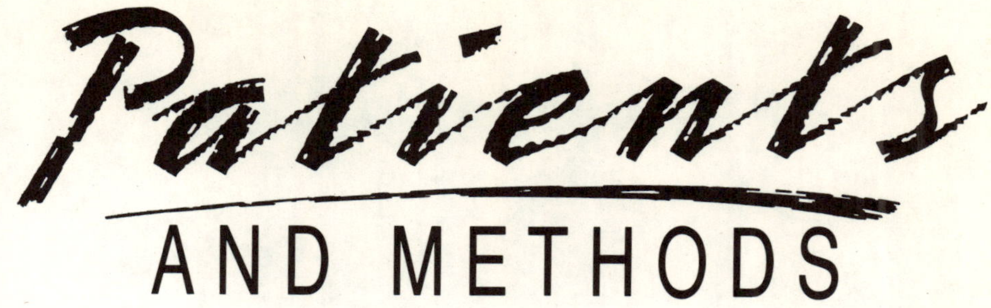

# AND METHODS

## CLINICAL METHODS APPLIED TO GENERAL PRACTICE

Douglas A. Gammon, *MBBS, FRACGP*

*Medical Director*
*Deer Park Community Health Centre*

*Senior Associate*
*Department of Community Medicine*
*University of Melbourne*

**McGRAW-HILL BOOK COMPANY Sydney**

New York St Louis San Francisco Auckland Bogotá
Caracas Hamburg Lisbon London Madrid Mexico Milan
Montreal New Delhi Oklahoma City Paris San Juan
São Paulo Singapore Tokyo Toronto

A52733

---

**National Library of Australia**
**Cataloguing-in-Publication data:**

Gammon, Douglas, A.
Patients and methods : clinical method applied to general practice.

Bibliography.
ISBN 0 07 452733 9.

1. Family medicine. 2. Medicine, Clinical. I. Title.

616

---

Produced in Australia by McGraw-Hill Book Company Australia Pty Limited
4 Barcoo Street, Roseville, NSW 2069
Typeset in Australia by Ku-ring-gai Typesetting Services
Printed in Hong Kong by Dah Hua Printing Press Co. Ltd

Sponsoring Editor: Lindsay Costelloe
Production Editor: Robert Paratore
Designer: Wing Ping Tong
Cover Illustrator: Patrice Guilbert
Illustrator: Diane Booth

To my wife Marie
for her support

# Contents

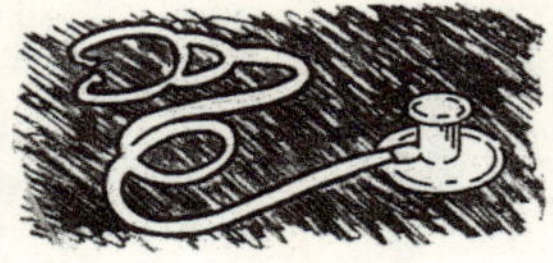

# Preface

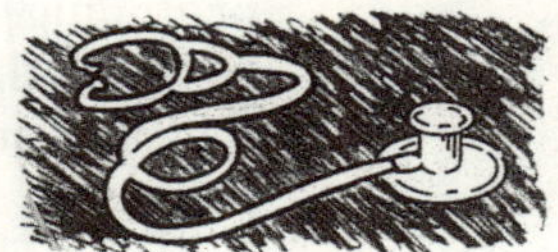

There is a gulf between hospital and general practice, and a corresponding gap in clinical texts, none of which describe a clinical method specifically designed for general practice. This book is intended to fill the gap by assisting those new to general practice to modify their hospital clinical method.

The importance of good clinical method is difficult to exaggerate, because significant consequences flow from general practice consultations.

Consider what happens when a patient is seen by a competent general practitioner. A highly skilled doctor, who sees an ill patient, makes a correct diagnosis and gives effective treatment leading to cure of the illness, is providing a very efficient and cost-effective service. Any illness that *can* be safely treated in general practice *is* treated in general practice.

When investigations are needed, they are intelligently and sparingly chosen. This limits the cost to the patient and the community. Good judgment is likewise applied by the highly skilled doctor when referral is required to the high-cost areas of specialist or hospital care. Thus general practitioner efficiency has a crucial influence on the whole health care system. Central to the efficiency is good clinical method.

In those new to general practice, responses vary: referring many patients to hospitals or specialists, over-investigating patients to bolster lack of confidence, and/or thoroughly examining every patient instead of exercising judgment and selection. Such responses relate more to a doctor's inability to tolerate the responsibility of first-contact care than to a patient's situation.

Responsible and efficient general practice depends on good clinical judgment based on systematic application of clinical method as outlined in this book: a blend of the human and the scientific.

There are some important disclaimers required about what the book does *not* aim to do:

- It does not aim to replace standard clinical texts, but to supplement them.
- It does not aim to teach treatment of specific diseases.
- It does not aim to teach 'in-depth' counselling of psychological illness.

It is concerned with clinical process and method in general practice. Experienced general practitioners may find in it little, if anything, new to them. But the overriding importance of good clinical method in general practice and the lack of a suitable clinical text provided the impulse for the book to be written.

The author has practised seventeen years in the inner city, fourteen years in the outer city, two years in the country and two years in hospital in Australia. Also, he has worked six months in general practice and one year in hospital in the UK.

His teaching experience consists of some eight years' clinical teaching in the inner city and twelve years' clinical and group teaching in the outer city practice. In that twelve years, some five hundred medical students and fifty Family Medicine Program doctors have gained experience in the practice. The author also had students attached to him both in hospital and general practice in the UK.

### Aims of the book

This book aims:

- to make doctors and students aware of the patient's total communication;
- to make students and young doctors aware that general practice is no less 'scientific' and intellectually demanding than hospital or specialist practice;
- to provide information about the nature of general practice;
- to emphasise the need for general practice to be based on critical evaluation of evidence.

### How to use this book

By students, it would be best read at the time of first introduction to hospital clinical practice so that they become aware of the differences between the two clinical worlds from the beginning of their clinical experience.

It should also be read again just before and during first student contact with clinical general practice.

By young graduates, it would be best read just before their first general practice attachment.

The cases quoted can be used as the basis for discussion by students or young graduates, singly with their clinical teacher or in groups.

By experienced doctors, it can be read at any time when they wish to review their clinical practice.

# Acknowledgments

The advice, suggestions and criticism of the following colleagues who read the manuscript are gratefully acknowledged: Dr Peter Rankin, Dr David Gome, Dr Therese Paulson, Dr Fiona Broderick, Dr Jacinta Opie, Dr Joanna Flynn and Professor Ross Webster. I thank my wife Marie and daughters Juliet and Cynthia and son Timothy for their support and encouragement. My thanks are also due to Dr John Williams, my daughter Elizabeth and my son Nicholas for their help in preparing the manuscript.

# Introduction

*'For two or three days my head has been whizzing round; I drink a bit of wine and I don't do anything, but it still goes round. And what causes my headache? I didn't come for six weeks because I kept hoping it would go by itself. Then yesterday the dizziness came and I was afraid to drive the car.'*—Louis, aged 53 years.

*'I'm feeling old, I've got a "cold", pain in my back, pain in my head, pain in my chest, lost my appetite, not eating. I should have come to see you last year. I lost my wife suddenly on the first of June.'*—Richard, aged 50 years.

*'John's had a bad pain in his stomach; this is the third time he's had it.'*—Mother, bringing in her son, who is 7 years old, for an urgent unscheduled consultation.

All of these cases are fraught with dire possibilities. Louis could have a cerebral tumour, labyrinthitis, acoustic neuroma, or it might be all due to alcohol and his wine drinking. Or perhaps some other cause?

Has Richard just got a cold and is feeling a bit down or is there some more sinister cause?

And John: is he brewing an acute appendicitis? Should he be sent to hospital or has he some more innocent condition that can safely be treated at home?

These are a sample of the approximately three hundred and seventy different problems that regularly confront general practitioners. How to deal safely with them, within the time constraint, is the subject of this book.

In fact, the three presenting problems described above were all successfully managed initially by clinical method alone, with only urine investigations done in the surgery to assist the diagnostic process.

The central purpose of the book is to describe a comprehensive clinical method appropriate to the demands of general practice. The method is comprehensive and flexible, and a prime aim is to teach a reliable diagnostic method based on critical evaluation of evidence, in the belief that the quality of practice ultimately depends on correct diagnosis.

But clinical method must include the formation of a clinically effective relationship with the patient, and attention must be paid to the non-verbal communication, which is mostly about feelings and attitudes that determine relationships. If the relationship is deficient, the scientific medical aspect of the consultation is likely to come to naught.

Thus, in a consultation two processes are being carried on simultaneously: the scientific collection and evaluation of data from history and examination, followed by diagnostic processes, and the sending and receiving of non-verbal communication on which rapport is built, followed by the development of confidence and negotiation of an agreement about what action is to be taken.

Relationships differ in different places. In hospital, Sister in her starched uniform showing a new patient to the allotted bed may say, 'Take all your clothes off, put this gown on and get into bed', in a tone that brooks no disobedience. The person becomes a depersonalised patient, a body clothed only in a hospital gown for convenience of access.

In general practice, the approach must be very different. Patients are welcomed with a smile by the doctor and invited to a chair, and there is normally an exchange of greetings and perhaps some chat about everyday affairs. Then patients are invited to tell the doctor about the problem troubling them. The telling is encouraged by apt response and close attention.

The doctor constantly monitors the non-verbal communication from the patient and modifies the course of the consultation accordingly. History taking and examination are largely curtailed or expanded to conform with acceptance by the patient. On occasions there may be a need to insist, but only after adequate explanation of the reasons, and again, only if the patient eventually signals acceptance.

In hospital, most patients are captives; only the sturdiest souls get up and walk out. Not so in general practice. There, the patient can stand up and walk out at any moment. All of which underlines the fact that the doctor's skill in forming an effective relationship with the patient is every bit as important as scientific medical knowledge. Hence the importance given to interpersonal relations in the case discussions in this book.

As indicated in Figure I1.1, one of the major difficulties of general practice is that many patients present problems which are undiagnosable when first seen. They may later become diagnosable or may get better without ever being diagnosed. They may cross the 'diagnostic threshold' or resolve spontaneously with only symptomatic treatment.

The enormous range of presenting problems, the need to form a clinically effective relationship with every patient, and the undiagnosability of many presenting problems at first contact, together make good clinical method an imperative for good general practice.

A consultation is the beginning of the clinical process, so we take a close look at the processes of a consultation in the next section.

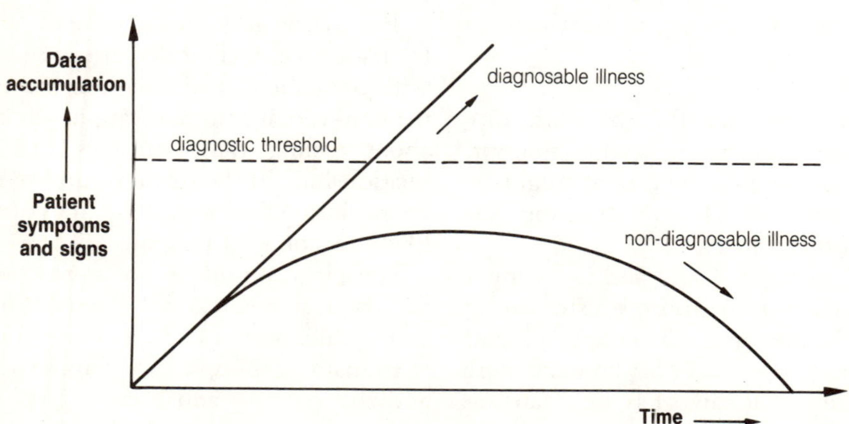


**Fig. I1.1** *Pathology is an evolving process that has a diagnostic threshold before which diagnosis is impossible. Diagnosis becomes possible when the necessary and sufficient evidence emerges. Many minor illnesses never reach the diagnostic threshold.*

# 1 Processes of a consultation

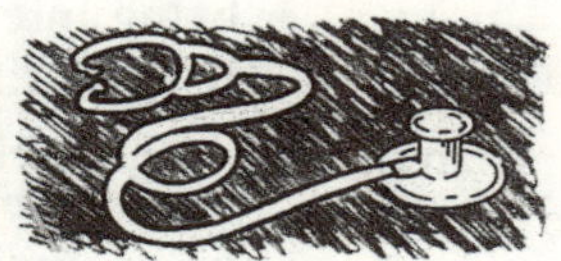

To understand what goes on in a consultation, it is useful to look at what each person does: doctor, patient and a third person. A third person is most often a parent, whose interactions with the doctor have been explored in Chapter 7.

Because the doctor is generally the pacesetter, we look first in detail at the doctor's activities, then at those of the patient, and lastly at the third person.

## What the doctor does

In a consultation, the doctor engages in data gathering, relationship generation and intellectual processes; to some extent these are all carried on concurrently, particularly in the early part of the consultation. We will look at each in turn.

## Data gathering

### The record

It is always a good idea to spend a few moments studying the record before you call the patient in.

Even with new patients, the record will provide you with some valuable information: marital status, age, occupation and possibly information gathered by nursing staff about past history and some details about the presenting complaint, including temperature, pulse rate, respiratory rate and blood pressure.

With an established patient, there will be much more information. Experienced doctors look first at the last entry, noting the date and whether it was recent or in the more distant past, the nature of the complaint, the outcome and what therapy was used. In a practice with a number of doctors, note will be taken of who saw the patient last and whether it was in or out of hours.

One of the things an experienced doctor does in looking at the record is to note the previous pattern of contacts. Patients tend to divide themselves into groups according to their ability to attach to a particular doctor. Some will only see their favourite, preferring to remain away when he or she is absent. Others will see two or three, out of four or five, but not the others. There is another group who will see whoever is most available, perhaps over a period seeing every doctor in the group without any apparent preference.

The RACGP record system used in the author's practice has a front-page summary of the most important medical facts about the patient. By studying this briefly, the doctor can rapidly become acquainted with the patient's past history. Past illnesses, family illnesses, social history, allergies to drugs or other substances and immunisation status are all recorded. At the back of the record there is a summary in chronological order of past investigations and reports about the patient (see Appendix 1—Records).

It happens at times that patients complain about certain symptoms at one consultation, and have

Forgotten all about them next time. Briefly record verbatim the patient's principal symptoms, so that at the next consultation, when they are worse or no better, one can jog their memories. The record then is an *aide-mémoire*.

### History taking

With patients new to the practice, it is best to take a full history and do a full regional examination, provided that this is acceptable to the patient. The data forms a 'baseline', and most patients will react well to being examined carefully; rapport and confidence will be strengthened.

Lack of time may not permit full history and examination, and then it may be best to say, 'I don't have time to go into this fully today; come back and see me again tomorrow and we'll go into it properly'. This is acceptable to most people unless there is urgency.

### Interview technique

Rather than going through a long series of direct questions, it is usually better for the patient to tell his or her own story as much as possible without direction. If one looks and sounds friendly, interested and concerned, the patient will be encouraged to tell more. There are several good examples of interview technique among the cases quoted.

### 'Open' questions

Usually the first question is an 'open' one, followed later by more closed questions to check on specific points. It is best to concentrate closely on everything the patient says, particularly early, then follow up clues and set out to generate rapport as rapidly as possible by non-verbal means.

Facilitating techniques can be used to encourage patients to reveal as much as possible of their story; direct closed questions tend to be threatening.

### Repetition

One such technique is to repeat something the patient said, avoiding any comment and adding nothing to it; simple repetition of the patient's statement is all that is required. This almost invariably stimulates the patient to enlarge and provide more information.

### Vocal responses

Varying the tone of voice is also important when using the above technique; perhaps sometimes being interrogatory and at others exclamatory. It is possible to develop quite a wide range of vocal responses, all devoid of any specific meaning but encouraging the patient to tell more in an undirected way.

Another technique is to comment on something about the patient, such as the way he or she walks, or moves, or looks, avoiding any question at all. This amounts to comment on some aspect of the patient's non-verbal communication. Again, the patient will usually respond by providing information relevant to the problem.

It is surprising at times how much information can be obtained by *not* asking questions. Again, there are examples in the cases quoted.

## General examination

### Illness

The first thing you notice about a patient is how 'ill' he or she is. The degree of illness determines whether there is urgency or not.

In the great majority of consultations, the patient walks in and sits down, and there is no urgency. But if Sister thumps on your door, runs in and asks you to come and see a patient straight away, you would be wise to respond to her assessment of urgency with immediate action.

Urgent calls are best treated as urgent. In the majority of instances, anxiety levels on the part of relatives are disproportionately great. On the other hand, experienced general practitioners will all have seen some cases in which the reverse was true; namely, that the patient's clinical state was more serious than anxiety in friends or relatives suggested. It is safest to make your own estimate of 'illness'.

### Intelligence

You are not interested in the patients' academic potential, but rather in whether their intelligence is impaired by illness to the point where they are not able to co-operate effectively. Are they fully aware of their situation?

### Co-operation

Co-operation requires a perception by the patient of the need for help from the doctor and an emotional attitude of acceptance of help. He or she needs to be willing to work with the doctor to achieve a resolution of the problem.

### Expression

The patient's expression reflects emotional mood and attitude to the individual doctor.

### Build and weight

This includes obesity, wasting and oedema. Weigh the patient and write down the result, so that next time you will be able to weigh them again and be aware of the trend. If the patient is slim, fit and athletic, at once a whole range of problems are rendered extremely unlikely. If wasting or significant oedema are present, it is very probable that there is some serious pathology. In obese patients, clinical assessment is less precise; for example, estimation of blood pressure, location of apex beat and abdominal palpation.

### Posture and movement

If the patient is upright, walks in briskly with a free gait and is precise and deft in movement, neuro-musculo-skeletal problems immediately become unlikely.

If the patient limps in bent over and complaining of pain, has difficulty in getting undressed and onto the couch, difficulty in turning over on the couch, difficulty getting off it again and dressing, neuro-musculo-skeletal problems are almost certainly present.

### Personal space

Up to this point your observations are purely by inspection; from now on you require some physical contact with the patient, who must accept this invasion of personal space. Begin by feeling pulse, observing and estimating respiration, taking blood pressure and temperature; these are only marginally invasive.

### Temperature, pulse, respiration and blood pressure

By recording these quantitatively, you will establish a 'baseline' and detect high fever (which is not always obvious), arrhythmias and hypertension; these might otherwise escape notice. You will also get strong clues as to what is required in detailed regional examination.

### Skin

The presence of pallor, cyanosis (best seen in the tongue), jaundice or abnormal pigmentation, rash and hair distribution provide further clues as to how regional examination should proceed.

### Swellings

Swellings are very varied and include skin lesions such as hives, insect bites, urticaria, boils, lipomas and sebaceous cysts. Breast lumps, enlarged lymph glands in cervical and inguinal regions, enlarged thyroid, bone cysts or other bone tumours and even oedema of the ankles may present in this way. The list is very extensive and includes a wide range of pathology.

### Deformities

Again, these can be very varied, including fractures, congenital conditions, minor irregularities of a baby's skull, or minor deformities of a young child's legs or feet. These are often brought to the doctor's attention by the patient or parent, but should always be sought.

In general examination, illness, intelligence, co-operation, expression, build and weight, posture and movement are all assessed very rapidly and often are completed by the time the patient has walked in, been greeted and shown to a chair. The process becomes almost automatic after some time in practice, but it is best to run through the checklist rapidly in your mind to avoid important omissions.

It is best to do it in full on all new patients, in follow-up consultations and consultations with regular patients. The only item that can be safely omitted in review is build; all others are susceptible to change.

If it is done systematically and routinely, the clinician is able to make rapid objective assessments of clinical state and use comparative pattern matching to accurately assess improvement or decline.

### Non-verbal communication from the patient

Data about emotions are communicated mainly non-verbally, and the doctor must be alert to pick up signals indicating anxiety, depression, anger, hostility, tiredness, boredom, friendliness, happiness or general wellbeing. The data that the doctor receives about the patient's emotional attitude is of equal importance with that from the patient's history and general examination in determining how the rest of the consultation must be conducted.

### Personal space data

Patients send signals to the doctor by their choice of chair; whether they opt to sit closer or farther away from the doctor. Initially, the majority choose the more distant chair, and occasionally a patient may take it on him or herself to rearrange the doctor's furniture by moving a chair much farther away behind the desk. Some come and sit close to the doctor from the beginning. Later in the consultation, most will move closer to permit the physical contact entailed in taking a blood pressure reading and other examination. Some then resume their original situation, others remain close. Choice of closeness by patients seems not to be related to sex; some men and some women adopting both courses of action.

### Psychological state checklist

This provides systematised data on the patient's mental state. At this point, if there is suggestive evidence of psychological illness, the doctor can run through rapidly in his or her mind the series of headings contained in the list (see Appendix 3—Clinical checklist).

### Regional examination

This is the same as is carried out in hospital, so it is not discussed in detail. Consult the 'Clinical checklist' at the end of the book if you wish to refresh your memory on any aspect.

What is different in general practice is the frequency with which it is carried out and what areas are examined; a clinical decision is made based on history, general examination and relationship as to what regional examination is necessary in each consultation. Acceptability to the patient depends on the relationship, which we will now consider.

## Relationship generation

In a consultation, the relationship that is formed between the doctor and patient goes through the phases of rapport development, generation of confidence by the patient in the doctor and, finally, negotiation of an agreement about management. The dominant influence, at least in the early stages, is the non-verbal communication that passes between them. So this will be considered a little further.

### Non-verbal communication to the patient

Facial expression is of prime importance; whether the patient is greeted with a smile, a neutral expression or a frown, whether appropriate eye contact is made, the tone of voice and the choice of words, all strongly influence the relationship with the patient. The doctor's bodily attitude, whether sitting forward in an attitude of close attention or leaning back less attentively, is important.

Seating arrangements send messages; if the doctor chooses to be separated from the patient by a desk or, instead, arranges for the patient to sit at right angles, closer, also influences the relationship.

Doctors send messages by their actions. An old person may be helped with dressing or undressing, or helped on or off the couch, indicating a caring attitude. So don't just sit there; do something.

### Rapport

Rapport is friendly, good feeling based on the doctor's caring attitude and the patient's desire for help. It governs the extent to which a patient will comply with advice; rapport is vital.

Rapport once formed with regular patients will endure for a while, but needs to be reinforced at every contact. One must appreciate the patient's problems and do something effective about them or at least be seen to be trying hard to help; friendly feeling alone is not enough.

Nothing generates rapport so quickly as effective relief of severe pain; for example, a digital block in a severely crushed index finger, or adequate morphine in severe chest pain.

Rapport can also be fostered by discussion of non-medical topics of common interest to both doctor and patient. More generally, showing close interest, concern and a willingness to help are the basic requirements.

### Confidence

Rapport is not enough by itself. The doctor must also generate confidence in the patient that he or she can help. To inspire confidence, the doctor must display confidence. The doctor's capability and knowledge must be evident to the patient. There must be willingness to listen to patients' ideas and to discuss problems together.

The degree to which patients want discussion with the doctor varies widely. Some patients come in and say, 'I'm crook, Doc; fix me up', or words to that effect. This is not based on stupidity, but on strong rapport and confidence built up in the past. Such people are delegating all decision making to the doctor, whom they know, like and trust. It tends to put the doctor on his or her mettle to do the best possible for the patient; the probability is that the doctor likes the patient, that they are friends.

At the other end of the spectrum are those patients who never stop querying what the doctor says, does and proposes. They want to know the reason for everything. They are likely to be intelligent, well informed and possibly tertiary educated. They are very easy to handle, if the doctor goes about it in the right fashion, and in the process much rapport and confidence in the doctor can be generated. In such cases, the doctor adopts a change of role to that of 'expert adviser', in place of that of 'the director', used with the first type of patient. Precise factual information is supplied in answer to every question and the alternatives for investigation and management are spelt out. The doctor can express an opinion as to the best course, but it is the patient who makes the decision. The doctor remains firmly in the role of 'expert adviser'.

Most patients, of course, fall somewhere between these two extremes, and one of the skills of general practice is in judging at what level of sophistication to talk to your patients.

So confidence in the doctor is built partly on a basis of rapport from past contacts, partly on the doctor's attitude of confidence and display of knowledge, and on meaningful discussion with the patient.

### Agreement

Before you can treat your patient, you have to negotiate an agreement with him or her. It may be a tacit agreement, invisible to the medical student sitting in, but it is nonetheless real. In such cases, it is based on what the doctor knows will be acceptable to the patient. Care is taken that what is proposed falls within the patient's expectations. If it did not, there would be rapid protest.

In the majority of cases, there is a real discussion and some process of negotiation, with the doctor suggesting various alternatives to find out the patient's reactions. These options have to be meaningfully discussed, with the doctor listening carefully to what the patient says.

Usually, patients have very valid reasons based on their social situation for the objections they raise. To be accepted, a proposal has to fit in with the patient's commitments to family, spouse and children, and any special requirements that may exist, and with commitment to employment.

Sometimes patients reluctantly accept advice that is contrary to their expectations, and sometimes agreement is not possible when a patient demands something which the doctor believes is not in the patient's best interests; then, if persuasion fails, refusal by the doctor must follow.

## Intellectual processes

Intellectual processes carried out in a medical consultation are critical assessment of data, summarising clinical evidence, carrying out diagnostic processes on the data collected, formation of a management plan and making a succession of clinical decisions.

### Critical assessment

All data collected by the doctor must be subjected to critical assessment as to its reliability. This critical process is carried on throughout the consultation and must be applied to data from history, examination and relationship.

In the case of history taking, several techniques have already been mentioned; those of asking 'open' questions, comment on some of the patient's non-verbal communication, and variation in tone of voice and facial expression by the doctor, all of which have the object of allowing the patient to tell more without being influenced by questions. They seek to ensure that what the patient tells is a true reflection of the problem troubling the patient.

Another technique is to ask increasingly 'closed' direct questions when the doctor perceives the need to check on something the patient has told.

Similar tactics may be needed in other history taking from time to time, but must be deployed with discretion. Non-verbal communication in the course of the interview is the guide as to how much critical assessment the patient will accept.

In history taking, the attitude should be never to believe what the patient tells, and never to disbelieve it; instead, search should be made for some other evidence to confirm or refute it.

Consistency is the principal test. What the doctor is told should be consistent with the whole body of knowledge about the patient, including the past history in the record. It should not be self-contradictory, should not be contradicted by a close relative and should be consistent with examination findings. Any apparent contradiction should lead to close scrutiny of the data.

Examination findings also need to be critically assessed. There is scope for a good deal of observer error in recordings of temperature, pulse, respiration and blood pressure. These are often recorded by the nurse initially, but you can recheck them both at the beginning and end of the consultation. They can also, of course, be checked at serial consultations.

The location of pain and tenderness needs to be checked several times to ensure valid results, and it is necessary to make quite sure that the patient understands the distinction between pain and tenderness. Time spent in making the distinction clear will not be wasted.

Critical assessment also extends to interpersonal relations with patients, as these strongly influence management.

### Summary of clinical evidence

The doctor makes a mental summary of the symptoms and signs and non-verbal data that have been collected and subjects them to a further critical review process. This review process is one of assessing each item of data and giving it a weighting in comparison with other items. Some items carry more weight in the diagnostic process than others.

For example, Koplik spots are decisive in a case with a febrile catarrhal illness and a rash. The finding of a large number of pus cells in a micro urine on a midstream specimen carries a greater weight in diagnosis than a symptom such as increased frequency of micturition. Generally, objective evidence which the doctor has been able to observe personally carries greater weight than symptoms.

### Diagnostic processes

The data, having been collected, critically assessed, summarised and reviewed, then must be subjected to the diagnostic process. Pattern matching, hypothesis generation and testing, probability and exclusion are all employed in the diagnostic method. Also, in some cases the first diagnosis is one of urgency. A social diagnosis is always important.

These processes have all been applied to each of the cases presented as an exercise to illustrate their relative importance.

### Pattern matching

This is the most common method and it is used in two different ways.

In the first method, the doctor matches the pattern of evidence in the summary with his or her mental image of a particular disease and makes a diagnosis on the closeness of the match.

In the second method, there is a matching process involving comparison between the pattern the patient currently presents and that presented at the previous contact. It is used in review of acute conditions over a period of days, and in regular patients with chronic disease over months or years.

This use of pattern matching to assess progress is one of the major reasons why doctor–patient continuity is so important; the other very important reasons are the doctor–patient relationship and the regular doctor's knowledge of the patient's problems.

The cases quoted contain examples of the use of pattern matching by both methods.

### Hypothesis generation and testing

This is the scientific method. A hypothesis is formed to explain the occurrence of symptoms and signs in terms of physical or psycho pathology. This hypothesis, or diagnosis, is then tested by one of several methods available in general practice.

To begin with, data can be sought by additional physical examination of the patient, or by laboratory or radiological investigations. The additional data is then examined to see whether it confirms or conflicts with the hypothesis.

Further, the hypothesis–diagnosis can be tested by treating the patient; for example, giving antibiotic therapy to a patient with possible bacterial infection. If the condition resolves, it strengthens the diagnosis, but not conclusively. The same result could occur if the condition were due to a virus not sensitive to antibiotics and the natural history of infection with the virus a brief five days; resolution is then inconclusive.

### Review

On occasions, review may be the only means of testing a hypothesis. In many cases of acute illness in young children in which a hypothesis of viral etiology is formed, the only practicable means of testing is by review the next day. Then the clinical state may tend to confirm the hypothesis or refute it.

In general practice, one of the most dangerous traps is due to the fact that when a serious, potentially killing disease is seen very early in its evolution, diagnosis may be impossible because the necessary and sufficient evidence needed is not available. Such cases are randomly distributed among mild, self-limiting illnesses and may be quite indistinguishable from them. Only by appropriate review can this very dangerous 'trap' be avoided.

### Probability

There is a strong element of probability in most diagnoses in general practice, and this method is very often combined with pattern matching. A pattern of data presents to the doctor, who judges largely on the basis of past experience what the chances are of a particular diagnosis. Further action is based on this probability, or at least strongly influenced by it.

Many mild, short-lived illnesses occur and are assumed, because of the pattern they present, to be due to viral infection. It is practically never possible to isolate the virus because the mildness of the illness, its short life span and cost preclude investigation and precise diagnosis.

A similar situation exists with many other mild, short-lived illnesses in which the patient has symptoms only for a short period. The patient quickly gets better, perhaps with symptomatic treatment, and the opportunity never occurs for precise diagnosis.

Thus pathology is a continuously evolving process with a diagnostic threshold that is quite often never reached (see Figure I1.1 on page xii). Data, or evidence, accumulates over a period of time until the necessary and sufficient evidence needed for a diagnosis is available; before then it is impossible.

### Exclusion

Safety requires that potentially lethal pathology be excluded as far a practicable. The doctor will consider what the probabilities and possibilities are and seek to exclude dangerous pathology by scrutinising and checking relevant parts of the history, seeking additional information and repeating parts of the examination to check the consistency of the findings.

Cerebrovascular accidents are not often a diagnostic problem and may be excluded by absence of disturbance of consciousness and normal physical signs, meningitis by absence of neck stiffness and Kernig's sign. On the other hand, cerebral tumour may not be excluded on normal physical signs, and referral and specialised investigation are necessary when there is doubt.

Cases of asthma that respond incompletely to therapy may require urgent referral. Patients with signs suggestive of pneumothorax or consolidation of lung may need to be referred more or less urgently, depending on the degree of illness of the patient.

Apart from acute life-threatening conditions, carcinoma and tuberculosis may need to be excluded by appropriate investigations and review.

Cardiac infarction due to coronary disease is the most common condition that needs to be excluded in cases presenting with chest pain. Exclusion rests on making a positive diagnosis of another condition in some cases, and on ECG and cardiac enzyme evidence in others; when the condition cannot be excluded, the patient should be offered referral to hospital.

Abdominal pain is a symptom of a wide range of pathological states; it is very common, and the prime concern is to exclude from home-management patients with a potentially lethal condition. When it is associated with vomiting, urgency compels referral to hospital if acute surgical conditions cannot be excluded with certainty.

Skin rashes characterised by petechial or blotchy features may be due to bacterial septicaemia or leukaemia and should be referred to hospital for exclusion of these conditions when first seen: time may be important and should not be wasted.

'Exclusion' in general practice often becomes a process of dividing cases that can be safely treated at home from those where safety demands management in hospital. When there is doubt, early review with comprehensive examination of the patient from head to toe, supported by critical assessment of the evidence, is the most reliable method.

### Social diagnosis

How will this illness affect, and be affected by, the patient's family, work or leisure pursuits? The answer is the social diagnosis.

The social diagnosis is always important. When it remains in the background and appears to be of little importance, probably the reason is that the patient's relationships are functioning well. However, if the illness puts undue stress on the social relationships, they may quickly come to the fore.

The doctor needs to be aware that denial of severe family difficulty is very common.

## What the patient does

Since there is a constant interaction between patient and doctor in the interview, there is a patient counterpart to most of the processes gone through by the doctor. The patient communicates data both verbally and non-verbally, generates a relationship, engages in critical assessment and makes decisions.

### Data communication

Verbally, the patient outlines the problem in terms of symptoms. Patients are usually led by the doctor's questions, but begin by communicating what is uppermost in mind. They don't tell all; they are prompted and reminded by questions, but decide themselves how much to tell. Some matters are consciously concealed and answers are given at times that the patient knows very well are untrue. The reasons for concealment are many, but one of the most important is that the truth is too painful.

Non-verbally, the patient communicates vital data to the doctor in every consultation. The communication is nearly always about feelings, whether the patient feels comfortable with the doctor or not, feels friendly or hostile; feelings determine how much is told.

### Relationship generation

Most patients quite deliberately set out to establish a friendly relationship with the doctor. They smile in answer to the doctor's greeting and might make some general remark such as, 'I haven't seen you for a long time' or 'Did you enjoy your holiday?' if the doctor has been away. They might also say, 'I waited until you came back' or mention with a hint of apology that they had to see someone else while the doctor was away. They make conversation of a general nature and the overall thrust of all of this is to make the doctor feel wanted and valued. They, too, work at generating rapport.

A minority of patients are abrasive in their behaviour and destructive of rapport.

### Critical assessment

The extent to which the patient exercises critical assessment varies widely from the tertiary-educated, well-informed patient to the other end of the scale occupied by those who delegate all decision making to the doctor.

The first wants an adult–adult relationship with the doctor and the second a parent–child relationship.

Educated patients may ask endless questions, wanting to know the reason for everything the doctor does. They may ask why the doctor wants to know some items of apparently unrelated history, why he or she wants to examine them all over when their complaint is localised, why he or she suggests some investigation or treatment or referral.

The trusting patient, who delegates all decision making, usually does so because of long-standing rapport with the doctor, not because of lack of intelligence. However, if what is proposed does not fall within expectations, there will be questioning.

Most patients fall in between these two extremes and want to be informed about their condition and to participate in deciding what is to be done, but are willing to be guided by the doctor.

### Decision making

As do doctors, so do patients make a string of decisions during a consultation. They decide how much to tell, how much to be examined, what investigations they are willing to have done, whether a proposed referral is acceptable and whether to co-operate in a scheme of treatment.

### Negotiation

The days when the doctor was an authoritarian figure who ordained what patients should take, and do, and submit to, have largely vanished. Instead, the doctor must put the options to the patients for choice as to what is acceptable. The patients take some responsibility for their own treatment; they are treated as adults.

The patient is under pressure from the symptoms and has restricted choice in practice. Refusal to accept treatment means that the symptoms must be endured longer and perhaps another doctor must be consulted, and the whole process gone through again. Acceptance is easier and more convenient.

## What a third person does

A third person may be a spouse, son or daughter, other relative or a friend from next door or at work. What their relationship is to the patient is not particularly important, but what is very important is that the patient has a strong desire for their presence. They must be wanted.

Occasionally, patients attend under a certain duress from their spouse, usually a wife. They may present alone or under the watchful and supervisory eye of the spouse, who is determined that certain matters must be aired and cleared up.

Sometimes the ground is prepared beforehand by a phone call from the third person, who requests that the doctor do so and so. 'I know he won't tell you, so I just thought I'd give you a ring.' Or on occasions the sex roles may be reversed.

The doctor must tread warily in such circumstances because of the need to preserve confidentiality between spouses. People often assume wrongly that they have a right to know their spouse's medical history. They do not.

But in the majority of cases the interview is a three-way affair and there is no problem with confidentiality; often, the intervention and support of the spouse can be very helpful.

It can be especially helpful in supplying a close-up view of the patient in cases of psychological illness such as depression of insidious onset, when behaviour change may be apparent to someone who knows the patient very well but to no one else. The same may apply to the very early stages of psychotic illness.

Again, it is very helpful to have an independent view of some events; for example, when a patient has lost consciousness, possibly due to epilepsy. Then the third person can perform an invaluable role in supplying a description of what happened.

A third person inevitably strongly influences an interview by his or her presence, and it is nearly always desirable for the patient to be seen alone later, except in the case of a young child accompanied by a parent. Only by doing so can effective communication between doctor and patient be ensured. A consultation is essentially a meeting of two minds; it is for two only.

* * *

We now go on to consider management of illness.

# 2
# Patient management

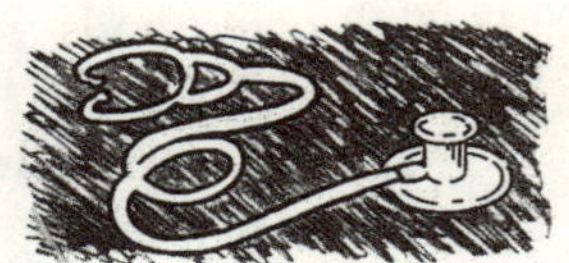

All of the following aspects may need to be considered when evolving a management plan for your patient.

### Investigation in the surgery

There is a range of chemical dip tests on urine that you can do yourself, and the results are immediately available. These include tests for protein, glucose, ketones, haemoglobin, bilirubin and urobilinogen; the manufacturer's literature contains details of sensitivity and reliability. Make sure your bottle of test strips has not passed its expiry date.

Also, it is valuable to be able to do micro urines and be confident about the findings. If you have to search to find a single cell in a drop of unspun urine, it is very unlikely that there will be active renal pathology. So a micro urine can be a very valuable negative screening test. The most important thing is to be able to identify red cells, pus cells and epithelial cells, and this is easily learned. If you feel the need, you can always check your positive urines by sending a sample to the laboratory.

A peak flow meter is essential to assess your asthma patients and is safer than relying on clinical assessment alone.

A Schiotz tonometer will permit you to detect chronic simple glaucoma.

### Laboratory investigations

In general practice, it is wise to order tests sparingly and rely more on clinical assessment and review, at least at the first consultation. It is essential to reach agreement with patients before ordering investigations.

On the other hand, many patients are strongly reassured by normal test results, which have a very definite therapeutic value. This applies to chest X-rays, electrocardiograms, serum cholesterol estimations and a range of other tests.

## Treatment

### To treat or not to treat?

This can be a very difficult question to answer. There must first be discussion with the patient about what action is to be taken, and this may involve quite prolonged explanation about whether treatment is necessary or not. There are many occasions when it may or may not be in the patient's best interests to treat a condition.

An example is that of a well, elderly patient with hypertension of 170/100. Such a condition is associated with an accelerated rate of atheroma development, which may lead to stroke. This risk has to be balanced against the possible development of symptoms due to antihypertensive therapy. Such symptoms tend to be more marked in the elderly, and symptoms have a large influence on compliance. Not many patients are likely to continue with therapy, especially for the rest of life, when the treatment makes them less well.

Much depends on how old the hypertensive patient is: 20 years, 30, 40, 50, 60, 70 or 80+. The potential benefits increase the younger the patient and the higher the blood pressure. The other factor is the patient's personality. Is he or she likely to comply with treatment or not? And for how long?

Acute viral infections are often treated with antibiotics, though there is little or no evidence of any secondary bacterial infection. The result is very often that there is some adverse reaction to the antibiotic, added to the viral illness, which runs its course in five days. If the patient gets a rash, this will probably be blamed on the antibiotic and possibly a note of false allergy to the drug recorded in the history.

Oedema of the ankles at the end of a hot day spent standing up is better managed by discussion and health education rather than oral diuretics.

## Discussion to educate

Education in the management of their own illness should be a part of your discussion with every patient, and the aim should be to give them as full an understanding as possible, both of the disease process and the treatment. The result will be greater compliance with therapy.

Patients are intensely interested in their own problems and are ideal subjects for health education. They are extremely receptive and have usually acquired some knowledge from the media on many topics. You, the doctor, are ideally placed to reinforce and increase their existing knowledge.

Patient understanding is very important in chronic diseases such as hypertension and diabetes mellitus, and the approach should be that the patient is the best person to manage the illness.

## Expectations

At this stage in the consultation, you should have a good idea as to the likely outcome of the illness and you should give the patient some idea of what time scale is involved—days, weeks or months. The patient must know what to expect.

## Counselling

Many patients prefer no drugs and will welcome alternatives. Anxiety may be much better treated by full discussion rather than by tranquillisers or sleeping tablets. If full information is provided and open discussion welcomed, the patient often responds very well.

## Counselling, health education and preventive care

Counselling, health education and preventive care are deservedly prominent features of modern-day general practice and are interwoven in the fabric of almost all consultations to some degree, but in differing proportions. There are examples in almost every case quoted.

## Previous drug therapy

The first point is whether the patient is allergic to any drug, or drugs, and detailed enquiry may be necessary to assess how reliable the 'allergy' may be. Usually, if there are alternatives readily available, a statement as to allergy is accepted at face value.

The next point to determine is what medication the patient is regularly taking and whether this has been medically or self initiated. Self medication of some degree is almost universal; it is rare to find someone who never takes a tablet of any sort. It is desirable in some cases to check up on self medication by asking for the tablets to be brought to you at the next contact, so that you know what the constituents are.

## New drug therapy

It is best to keep medication simple. Use as few tablets and as few doses as possible. Thus, drugs which require only one or two doses per day are preferred to those requiring three or four, because the compliance with less frequent dosage is much better. It is also better when the patient has only three or four bottles of tablets rather than six or eight. Compliance is best of all when there is only one bottle.

### Changing drug therapy

Be cautious about changing established therapy in patients new to you; changes should only be made for compelling reasons. If the patient is used to the regime, and stabilised, it is better to be slow about suggesting changes. Wait until you have seen the patient several times and have developed some rapport, then make your changes one at a time. The patient's regime has probably been arrived at by trial and error by the previous doctor and found to work for that particular patient.

### Avoiding tablet muddle

When a patient new to you is on an established regime of drug therapy, ask the patient to bring all his or her tablets to the next consultation. Then you can go through them together and avoid communication errors. It is very common for elderly patients to get into a muddle with their tablets, and this is to be avoided at all costs.

If you strongly suspect iatrogenic effects from existing medication, it may be best to stop all medication for a day, or two, or even three days, and see the patient each day until the effects have subsided. Then modified medication can be resumed.

### Treatment of symptoms

From the patient's viewpoint, the illness consists of the symptoms plus anxiety. Effective relief of both should be your primary aim.

Quite often, it is difficult to know which of a range of symptoms most need to be urgently relieved. The patient can be relied upon to tell you if you ask. Simply ask what is worrying them most and there will usually be a definite answer; then you know where to aim.

Very often, the primary need is to relieve the patient's worries. If you succeed in relieving anxiety, the patient will leave your surgery much happier than when he or she came in. Patients often say something like, 'I feel much better now that I've talked about it with you', and this is obviously supported by their non-verbal communication.

Anxiety is the main problem in chest pain not due to cardiac disease. There is, and has been, so much publicity about heart disease that anxiety about any chest pain is usually centred on the fear of a heart attack.

The best remedy is a full history and examination, to be followed by a chest X-ray, electrocardiogram, serum lipids and enzymes: when these are normal and the results are communicated to the patient, anxiety is largely dissipated.

### When to review a patient

The best guide on when to review a patient is when the relationship with that patient, or the pathology, demands it; most often there is a mix of these two reasons.

Patients who are acutely ill should be seen the next day or later the same day.

When you see an acutely ill patient before diagnosis is possible, don't say, 'If you're no better, come back in three days'. This demonstrates limited interest and concern by the doctor. Patients appreciate a much more positive approach. Say, 'I want to see you tomorrow. Make an appointment before you leave'. Be definite and directive. Patients never object to your taking an interest in them.

When asking patients to come back, tell them why; make it specific.

In the case of regular patients with chronic conditions, it is not always necessary to state explicitly why the patient should come back. Doctor and patient know each other's expectation. However, should there be a change in clinical state or therapy, then you should state definitely when and why you would like to see the patient again.

## Referral to local health workers

### Team care

Care of patients can be a team operation involving district nurses, physiotherapist, clinical psychologist and welfare counsellor. The team operation is of most value in cases such as alcoholism or schizophrenia, which affect all members of the family. Family situations are always complex and require a great deal of work and staff time if help is to be effective.

The most effective use of the team depends on the doctor having applied the clinical method correctly, having achieved a comprehensive assessment of physical pathology and a rapid survey of the psycho-socioeconomic problems surrounding the patient, and having formed a clinically effective relationship with the patient.

Then the doctor refers the patient to one of the team; which member depends on the nature of the problem, and on rapport. All team members must generate effective rapport if patients are to derive benefit. The team member then can explore the problem in depth.

### Communication

Communication begins at referral, ideally in face-to-face discussion between doctor and team member, or by telephone or letter. Plans are formed and agreed to by both team members, and details of implementation worked out. All of this is much easier in a health centre situation where workers are all in the same building. In other situations, a mutually agreed meeting time and place is valuable.

### Case conference

In complicated family situations, when several members of the family have been seen by different members of the team, a meeting of the team to exchange information and plan co-ordinated care is of great value.

### Clinical psychologist

The clinical psychologist is specially skilled in interview techniques and may spend up to an hour and a half with a new patient, supplying valuable assessment of patients with mental health problems and, in therapy, providing an alternative to drugs.

The clinical psychologist is of value in psychoneuroses, in marital counselling, in family relationship problems and in problems with children at school. In all of these, assessment and counselling can be of great help to the doctor and patient.

### District nurse

If the patient is confined to the home, the doctor usually makes a home visit and arranges with the district nurse to do follow up. Or on occasions when work load is heavy, the nurse does the first visit and reports to the doctor, and together they agree on further management.

District nurses are a vital part of the team and make regular visits to patients in their homes, in the process generating strong rapport with patient and family. They then become a very valuable additional source of information and advice about management.

### Physiotherapist

A physiotherapist provides valuable care in neuro-musculo-skeletal conditions. The physiotherapist is vital in acute stroke patients, for whom the potential benefits are very great. Pain relief, as an alternative to medication, is of great value to patients with chronic painful conditions such as arthritis or injuries. Restoration of function following injuries, or in arthritics or respiratory conditions, is a part of the physiotherapist's role. Adolescents with postural problems can respond dramatically.

### Welfare officer

A welfare counsellor can provide valuable service to patients in advising them about socioeconomic difficulties and can act as an advocate on their behalf in negotiations with various agencies when the patient is unable to state his or her case effectively. Emergency aid or accommodation can be arranged in crisis situations. The welfare officer may also be able to help resolve family problems by counselling. As with all the workers in the team, it depends on skill in generating rapport, and experience.

Referral to all of these workers requires the doctor to apply the clinical method correctly so that precise and accurate information can be supplied to the worker concerned, and a specific request made about the nature of the help required.

* * *

Referrals to medical specialists and hospitals are considered in the next section.

# 3
# Referrals

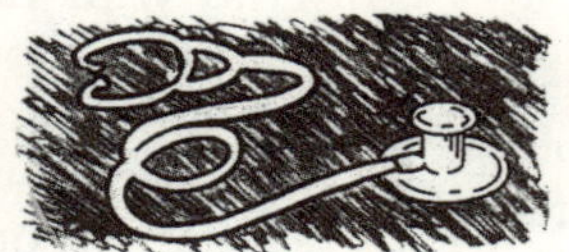

### Appropriate or inappropriate?

An appropriate referral can be of great benefit to the patient; less well-judged referrals may confer no benefit. Whether to refer a patient, and to which specialist or hospital, is one of the most important decisions the general practitioner makes for the patient.

### Cost

Any referral involves added cost to the patient perhaps in time lost from work and lost income, and some disruption of the patient's life and that of the family. As soon as a patient is referred, the monetary cost of the patient's care escalates very considerably and is ultimately a charge on the community.

### Outcome

The outcome of the referral is important to the general practitioner as it affects the relationship with the patient. After a successful referral that benefits the patient considerably, there will be considerable patient gratitude; after an unsuccessful referral, the reverse is the case. So it is important to all parties that referrals be well judged. It is a fact that all experienced general practitioners have a list of specialists to whom they regularly refer patients. These lists are constructed on the basis of the outcomes of past referrals.

## Initiative for referral

Referrals may have their origin in the patient, the general practitioner or a third party, who may be a spouse, a parent, work or leisure associate or even a friendly neighbour. Patients injured at work are often referred at the request of the employer, or an insurance company, or a solicitor consulted by the patient.

## Patient-generated referrals

Many patient requests for referral are very appropriate and may be for continuing treatment for some condition such as diabetic retinitis or glaucoma, or some other condition requiring specialist care.

On other occasions, requests may be wildly inappropriate and the patient completely uninformed about the advisability of the referral. Sometimes the patient does not even know the field of the specialist to whom he or she is requesting referral. On such occasions provision of advice is essential, though not always effective in changing the patient's intention.

The latter type of request is usually the result of the working of the local 'word of mouth' network, which often is very ill informed. Every community has a local 'word of mouth' network, which consists of relatives and friends, neighbours near the patient's home, associates at work or a local shopkeeper known to the patient. Advice is usually on the basis that 'someone else had exactly the same trouble' and it was 'completely cured' by going to see a named practitioner. It is notable that such advice is very strongly influential, though its rational basis is extremely tenuous.

## Doctor-generated referrals

The increased availability of pathology and radiology has provided the general practitioner with the opportunity to practise high quality scientific medicine. A competent general practitioner should be able to manage the majority of non-urgent patients with the aid of the diagnostic facilities available and there should always be adequate clinical assessment and investigation before referral.

Doctor-initiated referrals are sometimes for diagnostic reasons including highly specialised investigations, for overall assessment as to suitability for certain therapy, sometimes for specialised treatment, and perhaps most often for reasons to do with doctor–patient confidence. Persistent or recurrent pain that does not quickly abate is a prime reason for referral.

Specialised investigations include assessment of the suitability of a patient with angina for coronary bypass surgery. This is a good example of a referral that can be of very great benefit to the patient. There are also specialised investigations, including endoscopy in its varied forms, and scanning procedures, which likewise can be of great benefit, and the general practitioner needs to be aware of these advances.

### Urgency

Urgency often dictates what investigation is possible before referral, and on occasions it is best to refer the patient immediately. Urgent referrals may have to be done hurriedly, and in adverse circumstances, but the doctor should make every effort to communicate adequate data to the hospital medical staff who will be responsible for management.

Especially should the time, dose and nature of any injection be communicated, even in the most urgent circumstances. In less urgent cases, a record of past investigations and therapy should be included along with salient points of history and examination.

### Defective relationship

Doctors sometimes refer patients for reasons to do with rapport and confidence. Experienced general practitioners come to recognise patients who are going to do badly whatever therapy is embarked upon, and these people may be better referred sooner rather than later. It is better for the general practitioner to fail in company with the specialist than to fail alone. People who fall into this category may have personality characteristics that make it very difficult for any doctor to form an effective relationship with them.

## Third party-generated referrals

A case in point is that of a worker who has been injured and shows no progress towards recovery after perhaps four or five weeks. A request may be received from the employer or insurance company for the patient to be referred to a specialist. Such patients are best referred forthwith.

### Illness behaviour

Experienced general practitioners recognise two different patterns of response to injury. There are the majority who make steady progress towards recovery from the second consultation and a minority group who make little or no progress at all and whose symptoms get worse with the progress of time. As mentioned previously, they should be referred before illness behaviour becomes too entrenched.

Referrals may also be requested by members of the patient's family or friends, and at times the general practitioner may be fully aware that little benefit is likely to rebound to the patient though he or she has to comply with the request that has been made.

## Patient welfare is paramount

When the doctor has a free decision, without pressures from any source, the interests of the patient should be paramount and referral made if there is a reasonable prospect of benefit to the patient.

## Mix of all three

Very often the reasons for referral are a mix of reasons from all three sources. The patient may request referral, the doctor want it too because of the need for more precise diagnosis, or because of the need for specialised technology in diagnosis or treatment, or because the doctor knows the patient is not going to do well. A relative of the patient or employer or insurance company may request it too; so there may be unanimity.

## Referral letters

Referral letters should contain name, age, address, history and examination details, results of investigations and what treatment has been given. There should be a specific request as to what the specialist is being asked to do and what the patient has been told about the condition. It is best if the letter is typed.

If comprehensive letters on this pattern are sent with the patient, it is very likely that an equally informative reply will be received. The better the communication between the general practitioner and the specialist or hospital, the better the patient care.

Because referral is so important, ten consecutive referred cases are considered in some detail.

The main features are set out in Table 3.1.

**Table 3.1** *Referrals*

| *Case* | *Patient* | *Problem* | *Referral initiative* | *Outcome* |
|---|---|---|---|---|
| *1* | *22 years female* | *diarrhoea* | *doctor* | *Colonoscopy diagnosed Krohn's disease. Controlled by therapy.* |
| *2* | *3-week-old male* | *request for circumcision* | *parent* | *Operation successful.* |
| *3* | *2-week-old male* | *tongue tie, umbilical hernia* | *parent* | *Operation successful.* |
| *4* | *73 years female* | *chest pain* | *doctor* | *Referred to hospital. Later discharged well.* |
| *5* | *29 years male* | *tumour on finger* | *doctor* | *Diagnosed pyogenic granuloma. Treated. Cured.* |
| *6* | *32 years male* | *rash on soles* | *doctor and patient* | *Diagnosed pitted keratolysis. Treatment commenced.* |
| *7* | *26 years female* | *painful wrist* | *doctor* | *No pathology diagnosed.* |
| *8* | *67 years male* | *diabetic* | *doctor and patient* | *Continuing therapy of diabetic retinitis.* |
| *9* | *19 years male* | *painful back* | *doctor and patient* | *Gradual resolution and return to work.* |
| *10* | *27 years male* | *acute allergy suspected* | *doctor* | *Allergen not identified, but resolution occurred.* |

*Source*: Deer Park Community Health Centre records.

## Discussion

Initiatives for referral came in half these cases from the doctor, who anticipated the need for specialist help.

In case 1, the patient had been treated by fat-free diet, kaolin and finally metronidazole with only temporary success so the doctor came to suspect some underlying pathology. Colonoscopy diagnosed Krohn's disease, or ulcerative colitis, differentiation not being possible at the time. This patient was referred against a background of strong rapport.

In case 4, that of the elderly woman with chest pain, the doctor took charge and referred the patient to hospital entirely on his own initiative. This is the case entitled Ann and is considered in detail on pages 51–5.

Case 5 was that of a young man with a very vascular tumour of five weeks' duration located on the dorsum of his right index finger, about one centimetre in diameter and raised about half a centimetre from the skin surface. This was biopsied by the specialist, with considerable difficulty in arresting the haemorrhage, and proved to be a pyogenic granuloma. It was subsequently successfully removed.

Case 7 was that of a young woman with a painful wrist, which persisted over six months against a background of intermittent therapy and spasmodic attendance by the patient. There was no doctor–patient continuity in her management, and the doctor who decided to refer did so because she was making no progress. The referring doctor felt that every avenue should be explored, even though it was difficult to be optimistic in regard to the probable outcome.

The outcome was that no pathology was identified, and the patient ceased to attend for this condition though she did attend for other matters.

The remaining doctor-initiated referral, case 10, was a 27-year-old man with an acute generalised rash likely due to a chemical paint constituent with which he had come into contact at his work. With the object of precisely identifying the allergen, the doctor arranged for samples of all materials with which he had been working to be sent in to the specialist at the time of his consultation. But the test result did not indicate hypersensitivity to the material. The specialist advice was to treat the patient symptomatically for the present.

Of the cases referred by joint participation between doctor and patient, the 32-year-old man had a rash on his soles, which the doctor judged was due to his wearing safety boots at work and to excessive moisture. He had no symptoms from the condition, but was concerned about the appearance. Study of the record revealed that he had attended a year previously with the same complaint; there was unanimity about referral.

The outcome was the diagnosis of pitted keratolysis probably due to a corynebacterium or fungus. He was given antiperspirants and Whitfield's ointment, and this proved successful after six weeks.

The 19-year-old with the painful back had no abnormal signs and had attended intermittently with long absences. The doctor was convinced that the prospects of any effective therapy were poor, so he readily agreed to arrange the referral when the patient requested it.

The specialist considered that he had suffered significant trauma and advised rest and graduated return to work, which proved successful.

The 67-year-old man with diabetic retinitis was under continuing therapy from the ophthalmologist, and there was again unanimity about the need for referral.

The two young babies were both referred at the parents' request and against the inclination of the doctor, who felt that the operations were not really necessary.

In the first case the husband, who was seeking the operation, was not present and so there was no opportunity for discussion, but since husband and wife had reached agreement, the doctor made no attempt at dissuasion.

In the case of the mother of the second baby, she was very insistent that a referral should be made for the tongue tie and made no mention of the umbilical hernia, which it turned out was operated on at the same time.

In these last two cases, operation was performed successfully and there were no adverse effects.

# 4
# The time constraint

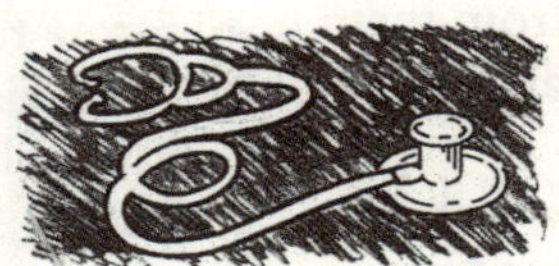

This section looks at the use of time in a general practice setting.

Enough time in a consultation must be given to arrive at a point of satisfaction to the patient; the patient's urgent concerns must be alleviated. The doctor cannot know how long the consultation will take before the event, and so appointment systems are often under some strain.

First consultations always take longer than reviews of the same patient. In a first consultation, the doctor must go through the full routine, cutting it down only on findings from general examination and non-verbal communication.

It is usually best to allocate time to take a full history and do a rapid head-to-toe examination with patients new to the practice. It is an efficient use of time.

Much of history taking is a once-only exercise and need not be done again. Once the data base is written into the history, it is there for future reference at all future contacts.

Again, it makes a favourable impression on patients if the doctor takes a full history and does a full examination, strongly tending to generate rapport and confidence.

Further, it provides the doctor with a baseline set of data against which the patient's progress can be checked; it permits effective monitoring of progress. And lastly, it provides full information on which to base diagnostic endeavours.

But with all these valid considerations in mind, one is forced back to the time constraint. It is simply not possible to go through a comprehensive clinical routine with every new complaint in general practice. One of the prime concerns of this book is to set out a safe method of abbreviating a full clinical routine; how to save time safely.

With new patients, if time does not permit the full deployment of the clinical method, it is often acceptable to the patient to say, 'I don't have time to go into this fully now; could we make a longer appointment tomorrow or whenever convenient?'.

Most patients will accept this because it demonstrates interest and concern by the doctor. It has a further advantage that it may result in further concerns coming to the forefront of the patient's mind; at the second session these can be ventilated.

Not all new patients require a lot of time; a result highly satisfactory to the patient can often be achieved quickly.

Review patients can usually be dealt with much more quickly, though success depends heavily on how they have been parted from at the first interview.

Patients should leave a consultation with a definite idea as to what they are required to do in the interim and why the doctor wants to see them again. The reasons for a further consultation should be spelled out.

Patients often recall only a very small amount of what has gone on in a consultation, and on occasions it is a good idea for the doctor to ask patients to repeat what they are required to do. Sometimes it may be necessary to go through it several times. Anxiety is a barrier to the reception and retention of what the doctor has said. The act of recall fixes it in the patient's mind.

When consultations are ended in this way, patients understand what is expected from them and why they should come back, and are usually happy to do so. When they are not, and there are two examples among the cases quoted, it is usually due to failure to generate an adequate relationship.

Review consultations can often be very brief and yet fulfil the patient's or parent's expectations extremely well. With acute viral illnesses, there may be a complete or almost complete resolution of the illness within a day or two. From being obviously ill one evening, a child may walk into the surgery next day almost well; or the process may take several days. Review by the doctor reinforces the parent's confidence; such reviews may last only four minutes.

Table 4.1 shows 106 consecutive consultations of one doctor and their duration.

A good many consultations were very brief and these were usually with patients wanting mainly a prescription or certificate, but also include a number of reviews of acute illness. These patients had usually been seen the previous day with an acute condition and had been asked to return to monitor progress and therapy.

**Table 4.1** *Duration of consultations*

| *Duration in minutes* | *During hours* | *After hours* |
|---|---|---|
| 0–4 | 18 | 0 |
| 5–9 | 31 | 10 |
| 10–14 | 18 | 10 |
| 15–19 | 6 | 3 |
| 20–24 | 3 | 1 |
| 25–29 | 2 | 0 |
| 30–34 | 2 | 0 |
| 35–39 | 1 | 0 |
| 40–44 | 0 | 0 |
| 45–49 | 0 | 0 |
| 50–54 | 0 | 1 |
| Total Patients | 81 | 25 |

*Source:* Deer Park Community Health Centre records

A few of the long consultations were due in part to the presence of students. The rest were new patients; some needed counselling about some psycho-social situation, and others needed procedures such as X-rays, application of plasters or suturing.

In the case of the consultation lasting 50–54 minutes, the patient had asthma and the time included history, examination and treatment with salbutamol, followed by a period of observation and counselling.

## Processes in time

*First minute*

### Relationship

Non-verbal communication flows between doctor and patient from the moment they set eyes on each other; rapport or anti-rapport commences.

The patient is welcomed and selects a chair in accordance with his or her needs for personal space.

### Data gathering

General examination—illness, intelligence, co-operation, expression, build and weight, posture and movement are noted at the same time as non-verbal communication.

History taking is commenced with the doctor noting the patient's presenting complaint and associated symptoms proffered by the patient.

### Intellectual processes

The doctor usually makes a rapid mental summary of the evidence at this point.

Critical assessment is made of the quality of the non-verbal communication, the likely significance of the symptoms, and a provisional diagnosis may be formed based on pattern matching.

In a known patient, the provisional diagnosis will rest on comparison of the presenting pattern with that presented at the last contact, or in a new patient on the closeness of fit between the doctor's mental image of a syndrome and that presented by the patient.

Rapid exclusion is made of life-threatening illness.

Clinical decisions are made about what questions to ask in response to the proffered symptoms and what responses to make in the light of the non-verbal communication from the patient.

At this stage the doctor usually encourages the patient to tell more by non-directive facilitating techniques. It is a good time to sit back and listen intently.

### *Second to fourth minutes*

#### Relationship

Non-verbal communication continues to and fro and rapport is becoming established more and more in the majority of instances; failure to develop rapport is also evident at this stage.

Towards the end of this stage personal space needs may be modified by the patient spontaneously moving closer or by invitation of the doctor.

By this time the patient's confidence in the doctor is growing.

Agreement is reached towards the end of the fourth minute as to how much the patient is to be examined.

#### Data gathering

History taking of the present state of health is largely completed and other relevant history taking embarked upon.

Temperature, pulse, respiration and blood pressure data are recorded, as well as skin characteristics of visible parts and presence or absence of oedema and swellings or deformities in most cases; some of these will be checked more completely later if the patient is undressed.

#### Intellectual processes

Critical assessment of the symptoms related by the patient is continued and some tests of validity applied, perhaps by direct questioning.

The doctor makes a revised mental summary of the evidence.

Provisional diagnosis is made now, based on pattern matching, probability and hypothesis generation, and testing perhaps tentatively embarked upon.

Clinical decisions are made to take past, family and social history in new patients or old patients with new complaints, and how much regional examination to do.

A decision is made as to how to present the doctor's perception of the problem to the patient, and this is immediately put into action.

Brief review consultations, and other brief consultations, end here with advice only, or a prescription and request for further review if needed.

Patients needing to be further examined are requested to remove clothing as necessary, shown to the couch, shown where to hang their clothes, given a sheet with which to cover themselves and screened by pulling the curtain across.

### *Fifth to ninth minutes*

#### Relationship

Non-verbal communication continues and rapport is strengthened as personal space between doctor and patient is reduced to zero by the doctor's physical contact with the patient during examination and the patient's acceptance of contact.

Patient confidence in the doctor continues to grow.

#### Data gathering

History taking is largely completed at this stage, but not infrequently various points may need to be confirmed by the doctor, and the patient often volunteers further information during examination.

Data on the patient's physical state is gathered by regional examination according to the schedule set out elsewhere in this book.

#### Intellectual processes

Critical assessment is made of data from history and examination by questioning and checking examination findings.

The doctor makes a further revised mental summary of the evidence.

Diagnostic processes include the full gamut of pattern matching, probability, hypothesis generation and testing, and exclusion.

Clinical decisions are made as to what, if any, investigations are required either in the surgery or by referral to diagnostic facilities.

The doctor makes a clinical decision as to how to present the medical view of the problem to the patient and what action needs to be taken. This view is then presented to the patient.

Many consultations end at this point with discussion leading to agreement as to the action to be taken.

After agreement is reached, the patient is given a prescription or advised that no drug therapy is required, is told when and why the doctor would like to see the patient again, and informed about necessary arrangements if referral is required.

### *Tenth to fourteenth minutes*

#### Relationship

Non-verbal communication continues and rapport grows stronger; negative rapport will probably have brought a consultation to a close by the end of nine minutes.

The patient will very likely reaffirm his or her need for personal space in the later stages of a consultation, even though rapport is very firm.

Quite extensive discussion may be necessary to explore and resolve patient anxieties at this stage and is usually the reason for the greater length of the consultation.

In terms of relationship, the aim of the discussion is the generation of confidence in the doctor and agreement as to what course of action to take.

#### Data gathering

This has usually been completed earlier, but additional material may be acquired during discussion as confidence grows.

#### Intellectual processes

Critical assessment of data is largely complete, though it will sometimes be modified in the light of additional material coming to light late in the consultation.

Again, there may need to be a revised mental summary of evidence with revised weighting of items of data.

Diagnostic processes mostly concern probability and hypothesis generation and testing; pattern matching and exclusion are used more in the shorter consultations.

Clinical decisions must be made about presentation of the medical view to the patient; presentation must be in a form suited to the patient if it is to gain acceptance. The doctor must talk at the right level in the right language.

Management decisions follow about drugs, investigations, referral and review. These must all be the subject of discussion and negotiation, leading to agreement between doctor and patient.

### *Last minute*

#### Relationship

Non-verbal communication continues with strong rapport and confidence evident in most cases. Personal space has ceased to be a concern.

#### Data gathering

Sometimes important data is communicated verbally to the doctor at this stage, either because the patient has overlooked it, or because of its sensitive nature. In the latter case, it may be that the patient has required the whole consultation to get to the point of disclosure, though this is distinctly uncommon in the author's experience.

Rarely, new data disclosed just before the end of the consultation may compel radical revision of the management plan.

What is not so uncommon is for the doctor to be uncertain just why the patient chose this time to consult. On the few occasions when it occurs, it is the author's practice to ask a direct question, 'Why did you come now?'.

### Intellectual processes

Critical assessment is virtually complete, but important clinical decisions are made about how to part from the patient. It is best to be strongly positive and definite about the diagnosis, and when the patient should be reviewed, and why.

Don't say, 'If you are no better come back next week', which is another way of saying, 'I don't know what's wrong with you and I hope to hell you'll be all right'.

Instead, even if you are in a hurry, say, 'I want to see you next Tuesday night to check your chest and make sure your bronchitis has cleared up', which is another way of saying, 'I'm interested in you, I'm concerned for your welfare, and I want you to get well; I care about you'.

# 5
# Adult cases

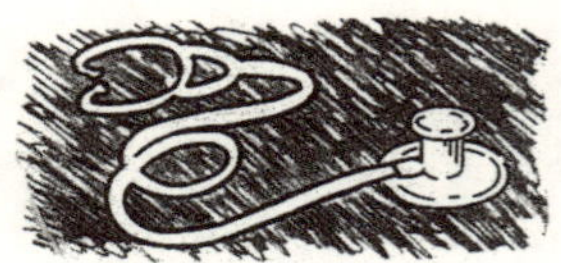

## Rob—episodic care consultation

### The record

Rob was a 21-year-old whose record showed he had attended three times in the last two years with minor viral illnesses. Five years ago he had had glandular fever and a year previously had been hospitalised with viral pneumonia. He was single and lived at home with his parents. There was no other information.

### Interview

DOCTOR How are you going?

ROB Oh not bad. I just found out tonight I've got a lump here on my leg. It's pretty sore. I found it when I was washing myself.

DOCTOR Do you feel well?

ROB Oh yes.

DOCTOR Got plenty of energy?

ROB Yes. I do a lot of running.

DOCTOR And you're running all right now?

ROB Yes.

DOCTOR I was just thinking that one of the possible causes is glandular fever and if you had that you wouldn't be able to run very well. But I see from your record you've already had that and you're not likely to get it again. So I'd better have a look at you and see if you've got a sore toe or something similar.

ROB I have got a sore toe. A blister that's got sore.

DOCTOR Well, that may be the cause. Let's have a look.

(*Inspection showed there was an obviously acutely inflamed blister on his big toe on the same side as the lump.*)

That's the cause of the lump. I'll give you some antibiotic that will fix the whole thing. But I want to test your urine and we should check your blood pressure.

ROB Oh great.

DOCTOR Take one of these tablets twice a day and it should clear up in a week.

ROB Oh! Just one more thing. I'm curious about a lump on my leg.

(*He displayed a minor swelling of a superficial vein at the site of junction with a deep communicating vein.*)

DOCTOR That's nothing to worry about. It's normal; everyone has them. It's just where two veins join.

ROB It usually pops up after my run.

DOCTOR When you've been running there is more blood flowing through it and that's why it pops up. There is no need to do anything to it at all. There you are (*handing the prescription to the patient*).

ROB Thanks.

DOCTOR Come and see me if the lump is not better after one week.

ROB OK.

## Interpersonal relations

### Non-verbal communication

The signals both sent to each other were friendly from the start. Both took to each other and felt at ease in each other's presence. Personal space was no problem for this patient, who came and sat next to the doctor.

### Rapport

This was established on a non-verbal basis and was reinforced because the doctor came straight to the point.

### Confidence

This seemed secure to the doctor because of the ease with which rapport had been generated.

### Agreement

The doctor perceived precisely what the patient wanted and provided it, so that there was no negotiation process.

## General examination

| | |
|---|---|
| *Illness* | Looked fit and well. |
| *Intelligence* | Good. |
| *Co-operation* | Excellent. |
| *Expression* | Good humoured. |
| *Build and weight* | Average, not obese. |
| *Posture and movement* | Upright, with quick precise movements. |
| *Temperature* | 37.0°C. |
| *Pulse* | 80 regular. |
| *Respiration* | Normal. |
| *Blood pressure* | 120/80. |
| *Skin* | No pallor, cyanosis, jaundice, pigmentation or rash; hair distribution normal. |
| *Swellings* | One on shin and one in left inguinal region |
| *Deformities* | Nil. |

On the basis of data from history, general examination and interpersonal relations, the doctor decided to limit regional examination to the legs. The patient was asked to remove both shoes, socks and his jeans.

## Summary of clinical evidence

He had noticed a painful lump in his left groin that day, but otherwise had been in his usual state of health, including his normal daily running activities.

He was a healthy young adult male of 21 years with an inflamed blister on his left big toe and enlarged tender lymph glands in the left inguinal region.

He was accustomed to run every day and reported that he was running well at present.

Urine examination was normal.

Rapport and confidence were strong.

## Diagnostic processes

### Pattern matching

The pattern of enlarged tender inguinal lymph glands associated with an acutely inflamed toe on the same side matched closely with the doctor's mental image of inguinal adenitis from a bacterial skin infection.

### Hypothesis generation and testing

The doctor formed the hypothesis that the patient had an adenitis of bacterial origin; this would be tested by treatment with antibiotics.

### Probability

The most likely cause of the symptoms and signs presented in an otherwise healthy young man was bacterial infection in the blister spreading to the lymph nodes in the inguinal region.

### Exclusion

*Lymphoma*

Glands enlarged by lymphoma are non-tender and there was likely to be diminished vitality.

*Infectious mononucleosus*

This was excluded by the patient's history of past infectious mononucleosus and his level of vitality.

*Lymphogranuloma venereum and syphilis*

These can be associated with unilateral inguinal lymph node enlargement but are extremely rare in the patient's community, no cases having been recorded in the last fourteen years. Again, the glands are not acutely tender.

### Provisional diagnosis

Inguinal adenitis secondary to bacterial infection in a blister.

### Social diagnosis

A young fit active man living at home.

## Management plan

Trimethoprim 80 mg + sulphamethoxazole 400 mg was prescribed to be taken after breakfast and the evening meal, the patient to be reviewed in one week if the condition were not completely resolved.

Duration of this consultation was six minutes.

The outcome was that the patient did not return until long afterwards, when he came for some unrelated condition and had forgotten about his sore lump.

## Discussion

The doctor began by asking an 'open' question, 'How are you going?'. This enabled the patient to say what he had come about, which he did succinctly and well. The doctor followed up with another 'open' question, 'Do you feel well?', to which the patient responded with a convincing 'Oh yes', leaving no doubt about it. Then a slightly more specific question, 'Got plenty of energy?', which elicited the response, 'Yes, I do a lot of running'.

And still the doctor pursued this question of general health and vitality; 'And you're running all right now?'. Again, a definite answer; a convincing 'Yes', with no hint of qualification.

With this assurance about the patient's general wellbeing, the doctor felt confident in limiting further history taking to the localised scene of the patient's left leg. The probability was very heavily that he was dealing with a purely local condition. So little more history was taken except as it bore directly on the local lesion.

Another very important aspect of focusing on the local lesion was that it conformed to the patient's expectations. He had come because he wanted to find out what the painful lump in his groin was and get it fixed up. So the doctor responded accordingly, and this direct approach had the effect of strongly generating rapport.

The rapport that was generated allowed the patient to mention another concern about the vein on his leg, which swelled after running; without strong rapport the patient may not have mentioned it.

This was a brief consultation lasting only six minutes and it illustrates clinical method applied in such a situation. The doctor took care to focus on the patient's concerns, while at the same time taking a history in such a way as to largely exclude serious underlying illness.

This was accomplished while fulfilling the patient's expectations and possibly answering some unasked questions. The main one of these unasked questions could be whether it had anything to do with glandular fever and whether his glandular fever had come back again.

Though rapid, the clinical method was comprehensive, with the doctor following a full general examination routine before deciding how to conduct the rest of the consultation. The decision to examine only the patient's lower extremities in detail was based on the data from the history, the relationship and the general examination findings.

But it should be noted that the doctor insisted on the patient removing jeans and both shoes and socks and comparing both legs by inspection. Almost invariably, patients proffer one limb for the doctor to diagnose, but one should always, always, always insist on sufficient undressing and comparison of both sides.

Had patient confidence appeared less secure to the doctor, or the patient more anxious, or the patient's general health and vitality less certain, full head-to-toe examination would have been carried out, reinforced by pathological investigations.

Follow-up would have been very important in this patient had treatment not been so effective, and very likely would have occurred because of the strong rapport. Clinically effective relations promote effective management.

★ ★ ★

Clinical method was applied selectively in this consultation to eliminate unnecessary history taking and regional examination, while meeting the patient's expectations and basic clinical requirements.

## Lilly—episodic care consultation

A consultation is a meeting of two minds; when the minds are not in tune, success is limited.

### The record

The patient, aged 35 years, had attended the clinic for eight years, in which she had been seen sixteen times, and her last attendance had been six months previously. She had blood pressure readings of 140/80 in 1980 and 140/90 in 1983. There had been two normal pregnancies and births in 1975 and 1980. She took the oral contraceptive pill and smoked six cigarettes per day. The only other illnesses had been minor viral infections.

The family record showed that her husband was aged 38 years and in good health, and that she had two sons aged 8 and 4 years of age.

Her father died aged 68 years of hypertension and cerebrovascular accident. There was no note about her mother. She had a sister who had asthma.

Lilly works full time as well as looking after the family. Her husband works regularly, but is an interstate truck driver and is away from home a good deal.

### Interview

DOCTOR How are you getting on?

LILLY Oh! Oh! Oh! I'm healthy enough, but these last few weeks I've been feeling so terribly exhausted and tired. I feel as though I just need a rest or something.

DOCTOR Are you working hard?

LILLY Oh yes! This is my problem. I work full time. I'm mother and father half the time. My husband goes away quite a lot. I'm just feeling a little bit drained at the moment.

DOCTOR Well you probably do need a rest.

LILLY I don't have anything wrong with me, but I just can't handle the situation any more. I get weepy. I'm getting like it now. They played a practical joke on me at work today and I just fell apart at the seams.

DOCTOR Are you sleeping?

LILLY My body is so tired that when I get into bed I can't switch off and relax. I have some good days when I race into work and watch TV at night, but when I get into bed I'm wide awake. And when I wake up in the morning at 4 o'clock I know I've got to get up at 5 o'clock. I just don't go back to sleep. And when it's time to get up at 5 o'clock I want to go to sleep.

DOCTOR How old are your boys?

LILLY One's 4 and the other's 8, nearly 9 years.

DOCTOR And they're both well?

LILLY Yes, my boys are well.

DOCTOR What about your husband?

LILLY He's an interstate driver.

DOCTOR And you're a widow while he's away!

LILLY *(with a laugh)* Well, yes. You could say that.

DOCTOR How long has he been doing that?

LILLY Oh! He's been a truck driver for years and years.

DOCTOR Have you ever discussed his getting a job closer?

LILLY Yes, we've talked about it. I said to him while I'm working full time there's really no need for him to be driving interstate as much as he does, but unfortunately his employers don't see it that way.

DOCTOR It would be better for you I'd imagine if he were home more to help with the children and jobs around the house.

LILLY He's very good when he's home; I'm just tired you know.

DOCTOR Well, you'd better have a week off.

LILLY (*with a laugh*) Oh goodness me! I don't know about a week. A few days maybe.

DOCTOR Well, I don't mind. I'm quite happy to write you out a certificate for a week if you want it.

LILLY Is there anything I could take to help me grab a few nights' total sleep? I'm sure that would pull me together.

DOCTOR Yes, it could help in the short term. You're just reacting to being over-tired.

LILLY I've discussed it with my husband and the reason that prompted me to come today is that I've been a bit volatile at home, forever screaming at the kids. And they played a practical joke on me at work today and I just went to pieces. I said to myself, 'This is no good, just no good.'

DOCTOR Are you quite well; everything's working all right?

LILLY Yes. Not so long ago I was checked over by my gynaecologist, who said everything was OK. She checked my blood pressure and said it should be watched, to keep an eye on it because it tends to get a little bit high from time to time.

DOCTOR Yes. There are two recordings in your record which are not too bad.

LILLY Do you want my jumper off?

DOCTOR Yes, If we're going to take it we'd better do it properly.

LILLY Is that all right? (*referring to the sleeve of her blouse*)

DOCTOR It's still a bit tight. You'd better take the blouse off too. You haven't had a cold lately, or a cough?

LILLY No.

DOCTOR Are your children all right?

LILLY Yes, my boys keep pretty good health.

DOCTOR There has been a small epidemic lately.

LILLY One of them was a bit weepy tonight and wanted to come to the doctor's with me, but I said, 'We'll see how you are tomorrow'.

DOCTOR Your pressure is a little bit up today, probably because you've had an upset day. We wouldn't pay much attention to this reading, but it is something you should keep an eye on. Have you lost any weight?

LILLY I haven't weighed myself lately, but I don't think so. I've always been a slim type.

DOCTOR Well, the best thing I can do to help is give you some tablets to sleep better and a certificate for three days. Have you ever taken anything to help you sleep?

LILLY Never! I don't like to start or make a habit of it, but . . .

DOCTOR But when you're working full time you have to get some sleep.

LILLY I promise myself some early nights, but when I go to bed I just don't sleep.

DOCTOR But you can't go to bed because you have the boys to look after. You have to spend a bit of time with them if you've got the energy. That's important.

LILLY Well, that's another thing. I thought while I'm feeling like this I could just have a rest at home and do that very thing, instead of racing them over to kinder and the grandparents and all the rest of it. It might make me feel a bit better inside.

DOCTOR You can't take a week off?

LILLY I don't like to. I don't take a lot of time off, but I know I've got about three or four days. If I don't feel any better by the weekend I'll come back.

DOCTOR All right. Have you ever taken tranquillisers?

LILLY No, but I know of them. My husband's been on them, but I've never taken them.

DOCTOR It might be better if I gave you sleeping tablets for you to take one at night about an hour before you go to bed. And we'll see how that works out. I'll give you a certificate for the rest of the week.

LILLY Yes, that'll be good because I'd like to keep some days in case the boys get sick and I have to stop home with them. I'll take the rest of the week and that'll give me a few good nights' sleep and make me feel better. Just one of these is it? (*referring to the sleeping tablets*)

DOCTOR Yes, about an hour before bed.

LILLY And my blood pressure's all right?

DOCTOR No, it's up a bit. Not much, but you're not such an old lady, so we should watch it. I would like to take it again in a few days.

LILLY All right. Thank you, doctor. If I don't feel any better by the weekend I'll come back.

## Interpersonal relations

### Non-verbal communication

The signals the doctor received were friendly but distant. There was an element of rigidity about her that was not susceptible to influence. This attitude remained throughout the interview despite the doctor's best efforts to be sympathetic and helpful. The doctor felt excluded by a barrier from meaningful contact.

### Rapport

This did not develop to any significant degree, though the doctor did all he could to generate rapport; the patient remained unresponsive.

### Confidence

The doctor felt this to be inadequate throughout.

### Agreement

There was no real agreement. The patient had a definite idea as to what she wanted the doctor to do for her, and refused to consider alternatives. The doctor wanted her to come back to have her blood pressure checked, but she would not agree to this. The interview ended with the doctor meeting her limited expectations, but failing to influence the outcome.

## General examination

| | |
|---|---|
| *Illness* | Not severely ill. |
| *Intelligence* | Average or above. |
| *Co-operation* | Limited. |
| *Expression* | Worn, tired and anxious. |
| *Build and weight* | Slim, but not wasted. |
| *Posture and movement* | Upright, moving a shade slowly, but precise and deft in her movements. |
| *Temperature* | 37.0°C. |
| *Pulse* | 80 regular. |
| *Respiration* | Normal. |
| *Blood pressure* | 170/100 seated after some four or five minutes of interview. |
| *Skin* | No pallor, cyanosis, jaundice, pigmentation, or rash; hair distribution appeared normal as far as could be ascertained in a fully dressed patient. |
| *Swellings* | Nil. |
| *Deformities* | Nil. |

The doctor made a clinical decision at this point not to suggest any further examination, as it was clear from non-verbal communication that this would not be welcome.

## Summary of clinical evidence

A woman of 35 years of age who presented because of emotional lability at home, manifested by screaming at the children and emotional upset at work with the other employees.

She lives a very stressful life with a full-time job, as well as her housekeeping and mothering roles, aggravated by frequent absence of her husband from the home.

She looked worn, anxious and tired, and had a blood pressure of 170/100 at this consultation, previous readings in 1980 of 140/80 and in 1983 of 140/90, history that her gynaecologist had mentioned her blood pressure as needing surveillance, and family history of hypertension.

Rapport and confidence were not at a clinically effective level.

## Diagnostic processes

### Pattern matching

The pattern of tiredness, anxiety, emotional lability and insomnia matched with the doctor's mental image of stress reaction due to overwork, anxiety state, or anxiety state superimposed on an underlying depression.

Blood pressure of 170/100 at this consultation, previous readings in 1980 of 140/80 and in 1983 of 140/90, and the history from the gynaecologist that her pressure needed watching, matched closely with the doctor's mental image of early hypertension.

## Hypothesis generation and testing

The doctor formed the hypothesis that the patient was suffering from stress reaction to overwork or anxiety with underlying depression, and early essential hypertension.

These hypotheses would be tested by prescribing sedative at night, providing the patient with a sick certificate for three days' rest from her work, and by subsequent review and investigation of both her mental state and blood pressure.

### Probability

In the doctor's judgment, the patient's pattern of psychological symptoms was most likely due to stress.

The blood pressure of 170/100 was probably due to early essential hypertension aggravated by stress.

### Exclusion

Depression should be excluded by review, possibly in a joint interview with her husband. The help of a clinical psychologist would be sought if acceptable.

Remediable causes for her hypertension could only be excluded by investigation.

### Provisional diagnosis

Stress reaction and early essential hypertension.

### Social diagnosis

A nuclear family of husband, wife and two young boys aged 4 years and 8 years of age, all at risk of emotional trauma, due to excessive social and economic stress on the mother. There is risk of complete family breakdown.

## Management plan

She was given nitrazepam 5 mg tablets to be taken one hour before bed, and a certificate for her to remain off work for three days.

The doctor planned early review and a joint interview with the patient and her husband if this could be arranged.

A range of investigations would be embarked upon relevant to her blood pressure if she wished to have these done.

The duration of this consultation was twenty minutes.

### Outcome

She did not return in the following week.

Subsequent search of her file showed that she returned after a lapse of two months in a similar state of minor crisis. She had broken down into tears at work, had a mild viral infection at the time and had been dry retching. She had been seen by a woman doctor, who had made a follow-up appointment for four days later, which again she did not keep.

## Discussion

This patient should obviously have investigations done relevant to her hypertension, as she was only 35 years of age and there was a family history of hypertensive troubles on her father's side. There should be scrutiny of her obstetric record, which purported to be trouble free, and there should be full clinical examination done, which was lacking at this consultation. It would be of value to seek a report from her gynaecologist as this might provide data about her obstetric record.

She should have had urine investigation done and, probably, in view of her age, should have an intravenous pyelogram to exclude renal causes of her hypertension. There should be haematological investigations, checking of her electrolytes and a chest X-ray as a minimum. Further investigations might be needed, depending on the outcome of these initial ones.

What of the patient's psychological state? We could look at her against the background of the Psychological State Checklist. This runs as follows:

General appearance and behaviour unremarkable.

Thought processes as judged from her talk were normal.

Mood exhibited some anxiety.

Delusions were not apparent.

Hallucinations were likewise absent.

Obsessions not present.

Her orientation was normal in space and time.

Memory was good.

Attention and concentration were normal.

General information fund appeared normal.

Insight and judgment were not obviously astray, though she may have lacked some insight into her relationship with her husband.

She had no obviously disturbed personality traits.

In summary, she presented as a tired, overstressed lady who was somewhat anxious, but not excessively so.

Was she depressed? She had sleep disturbance, sometimes having difficulty in going to sleep and sometimes early waking; she was tired, was tearful at times, but had no real depression of mood at the interview and had no weight loss or lack of energy. In fact, she was coping with a full-time job, housekeeping and mothering, and with a husband who was frequently away from home. In view of this evidence, a diagnosis of depression was difficult to sustain.

Rather than trying the patient on antidepressants in such a doubtful situation, the doctor opted to meet her request for a few nights' total sleep as he knew from experience that patients who are very short of sleep improve rapidly and considerably after one or two nights' sound sleep. Then the patient could be seen again and a reassessment made of the diagnosis.

An additional reason for not opting for a trial of antidepressant was the lack of rapport and her failure to comply with follow-up suggestions. Antidepressants are slow to work, and the patient must be willing to persist for a week or two before any benefit is seen. In this patient, the likelihood of such compliance was poor.

What other alternatives were open to the doctor? He could have refused to supply her with any sleeping tablets and suggested counselling instead, but did not do so because of the failure to develop rapport. He judged it very unlikely that she would be interested in counselling. To have refused her request for tablets would only have alienated her further and destroyed any hope of future co-operation.

The doctor whom she saw in this consultation wondered if she would react better to a woman doctor. She had referred to 'my gynaecologist' as 'she', but subsequent events at her next presentation when she was attended by a woman doctor gave the lie to this idea; the outcome was the same. She had been advised by her gynaecologist to get her blood pressure checked, but refused by her actions to do anything effective about the problem.

Another possible approach was to follow up through husband and children. A note could be made in each file to refer to the mother's file for information on the family when any of them attended. This would need to be very discreet in order not to breach confidentiality requirements between spouses.

The doctor perceived this lady and her family as being at risk of serious emotional harm should she break down and be unable to continue her central role. The whole family was obviously dependent on her. With this thought in mind, the doctor considered the possibility of a joint interview with both the patient and her husband as a first step in trying to devise some way of easing her burden. If this first step were achieved, possibly the assistance of the clinical psychologist could be enlisted to achieve an in-depth assessment of the family situation.

It was no surprise to the doctor when she did not return in the following week, as he had expected it from the failure of rapport to develop between them. This patient was accustomed to coming in a crisis, and seeing the first doctor available, but resisted efforts to follow up and achieve some lasting benefit. Study of her record revealed that she had seen every doctor in the practice, but never more than once for the same illness. It appeared that she kept all doctors at arm's length and failed to develop rapport with any one.

One wonders about her other relationships with her husband, children and work associates. She said her marriage and children were good, and healthy, but didn't go into any detail. She mentioned that one of the boys had been a bit weepy and wanted to come to the doctor with her, but her response was to say, 'We'll see how you are tomorrow'. Was she also emotionally distant with her children?

She had discussed her husband's job with him, but said there were barriers to any change. How real were those barriers? Or had they used the work situation to connive jointly at the existing situation? Did she really want her husband at home more? In short, how far are her problems of her own making? No answers are possible to these questions because of her determination to keep her distance.

In fact, much later, the doctor who saw the wife, also saw the husband. He presented with serious psychological problems of long standing. Was the wife engaging in denial? And why?

* * *

Clinical method was limited to history taking, together with some counselling, attempted relationship formation and general examination. The doctor perceived that more examination was unacceptable.

## Thomas—preventive care consultation

Preventive care is a feature of many consultations, but with this patient and family the potential benefits seemed unusually great.

### The record

Thomas, aged 45 years, was taking atenolol 100 mg mane for hypertension recorded as 170/100 two years before, and since then there had been readings of 170/110, 140/85, 160/100 and 160/110. His weight was recorded as 96.6 kg when first seen, but he had lost 6 kg after he had been advised to lose weight.

Apart from hypertension, his past history showed only that he had a fractured cheek corrected surgically eighteen years ago, that he had tetanus toxoid fourteen years ago and that he had no known allergies. He had had an intravenous pyelogram two years previously, which was reported as normal, and he had also had an ECG, but there was no record of the result.

He was employed as a clerk, did not smoke and drank six glasses of beer approximately per week. His wife was aged 45 years and he had two sons aged 18 years and 16 years.

Jennifer, his wife, also had had hypertension for twelve months and had been taking methyldopa 125 mg twice daily. She had a tubal ligation fourteen years ago, a tetanus toxoid injection fifteen years previously, was a non-smoker and had an occasional drink of alcoholic beverage socially. She had no known allergies.

James, aged 18 years, had asthma as a child, but this had ceased to be a problem; he was well, and a full-time student. He had had tetanus toxoid four years ago.

Ken was aged 16 years and had had a head injury eight years before, for which he had spent two days in hospital. He also had had tetanus toxoid four years previously. Neither of the boys smoked.

As regards the previous generation. Thomas's mother was alive and well, aged 60 years, but there was no information about his father. Jennifer's parents were both alive, aged 62 years and 65 years, and both had had a myocardial infarction. There was no other information available.

## First consultation

Thomas came to this consultation because he wanted his three-monthly blood pressure check and to get further supplies of tablets. He was feeling well, his pressure was found to be 160/110 and his urine test was normal.

He was given hydrochlorothiazide 50 mg + amiloride 5 mg compound tablets to take one mane as a supplement for his antihypertensive therapy.

Serum lipids, electrolytes and haemoglobin, packed cell volume, mean corpuscular haemoglobin concentration and a blood film were ordered, and it was arranged to see him again in two weeks.

## Second consultation

At this consultation his blood pressure was recorded as 160/110 at the first reading and 150/90 at the second one near the end of the consultation, when he and the doctor had been discussing at some length what should be done. Both readings were with the patient seated.

The haematological results were all within normal limits, as were the serum electrolytes.

Other results showed fasting cholesterol 6.2 mmol/l, HDL cholesterol 1.46 mmol/l, triglyceride 3.9 mmo/l, which was reported as elevated; the normal range was quoted as 0.2–1.8.

The doctor advised weight reduction, that the patient take regular daily physical exercise and that he should give some thought to changing his diet. It was suggested that the dietary change should be towards a more vegetarian one, with strict limitation of saturated fat and substitution of polyunsaturated fats and cooking oil, and limitation of calorie intake.

He was also advised to discuss life style and diet with his wife and boys, and was given some pamphlets with written advice and vegetarian recipes. It was pointed out that the whole family stood to benefit if they were able to make the suggested changes.

He was told that further investigations might be needed and was asked to attend again in two weeks, and that perhaps he might be able to bring the rest of the family too for a discussion.

## Discussion

If the hypertension were not better controlled at the next consultation, decisions would have to be made about possible changes to therapy and further investigation; probably a chest X-ray and ECG would be ordered and possibly other more specialised investigations later.

One of the major difficulties in treating patients with hypertension is that there may be no symptoms at all, as in this case, and the patient may find it hard to accept therapy or investigations. This patient fortunately presented as very co-operative, but the doctor decided not to launch into many investigations too quickly.

The potential for preventive care in this family was high as the boys were both young, and there is evidence that changing diet early in life confers considerable benefit.

Thomas showed evidence of motivation as he had lost 6 kg in weight earlier when advised to do so and he was taking his medication correctly and attending for review when requested; there was a pattern of compliance.

Finally, personal relations with the doctor were good with friendly non-verbal communication and rapport. When all of these aspects were considered, the doctor felt that there was a good chance of long-term benefit for the family.

The doctor hoped that if it were possible to have a family group discussion that it might aid co-operation with changes. Persuading people to change their way of living depends heavily on convincing them of the benefits. And the doctor saw it as sound counselling practice to involve the two adolescents in the discussion process.

A further alternative in management would be to involve the family as a group in a health education session; they could be put on the list of people to be invited.

* * *

Clinical method was confined to an open question about symptoms, formation of a clinically effective relationship, general examination and checking of blood pressure and urine. Full clinical method would be employed at the next review if the hypertension were not adequately controlled.

## Richard—continuing care consultation

This is the first of five consultations extending over as many weeks, but only two are described.

### First consultation

#### The record

Richard was aged 50 years. The doctor studied the record for a few moments before calling the patient in and noted that though the record extended over seven years they had never met. He had been an infrequent attender and had not attached himself to any individual doctor. There had been only minor illnesses except for one episode of indigestion investigated by barium meal. This reportedly showed a healed duodenal ulcer. The patient smoked twenty cigarettes per day and was a social drinker.

There was a strong family history of duodenal ulcer, both the patient's father and brother having had one.

His wife had died suddenly and unexpectedly the previous year, having been taken ill at work with a cerebral haemorrhage from which she never recovered consciousness despite urgent CAT scan and surgery.

He had a daughter aged 26 years, who was not a patient of the practice, and a son aged 21 years, who had had only minor illnesses.

He lived alone in his own home since his wife's death, and his daughter visited him almost daily. She was married with a young family in a neighbouring suburb. His son lived many kilometres away in a country town and had much less contact with his father. The patient had a long-standing safe job as a plumber and there was no record of any problems stemming from his work.

### Interview

DOCTOR How are you getting on?

RICHARD I'm feeling old. I've got a 'cold', pain in my chest, pain in my back, pain in my head. I should have come to see you last year. I lost my wife suddenly on the first of June last year. Lost my appetite, pains in my chest, not sleeping.

DOCTOR You've got a cold?

RICHARD Yes; for a while. I've had a cold for ages. It's shocking.

DOCTOR So you've had a cold for a few weeks and lost your appetite over a longer period. What sort of 'cold'?

RICHARD Oh! Coughing up phlegm every morning when I wake up.

DOCTOR What sort of stuff? What colour?

RICHARD Just phlegm. White.

DOCTOR Not yellow or green?

RICHARD No.

DOCTOR You're pretty sure?

RICHARD Well, it's mostly white.

DOCTOR And you're not sleeping? How long for?

RICHARD I wake up at 3.30 in the morning. I know I've tried going to bed at 12 o'clock and 1 o'clock. I tried going to the doctor. He gave me some tablets, but they didn't work.

DOCTOR Have you had any tummy upset? Vomiting or diarrhoea?

RICHARD Yes, I had diarrhoea.

DOCTOR Today?

RICHARD Yes.

DOCTOR How many times?

RICHARD Oh just once. Bowel is a bit loose sometimes. I'm very nervous as well. My daughter was worrying about me last night. When I'm asleep I jump.

DOCTOR Have you lost any weight?

RICHARD I think I have actually.

DOCTOR In the last twelve months?

RICHARD Well, I went for a holiday and stayed with relatives for three months, and I put on a stone, but I think I've lost it again.

DOCTOR Well, as compared with twelve months ago, would you say you've lost weight? You should be able to tell from your clothes. Are your clothes looser on you?

RICHARD I think I have actually.

DOCTOR And you lost your wife last year did you?

RICHARD She was working and they thought she had had a heart attack.

DOCTOR Yes, I remember she was brought round here and we sent her straight down to the hospital.

RICHARD She never regained consciousness.

DOCTOR Are you working?

RICHARD Yes.

DOCTOR Are you happy in the job?

RICHARD Oh! Yes.

DOCTOR I'd better look at you thoroughly. Would you take your clothes off?

RICHARD What exactly?

DOCTOR Take everything off except your underpants so I can have a quick run over you.

RICHARD I get cramp a lot.

DOCTOR At night?

RICHARD Anytime.

(*There followed a pause while the examination was done.*)

DOCTOR Put your clothes on before you get cold. And would you pass a specimen of urine for me?

(*The doctor dip-tested this while the patient finished getting dressed.*)

That was normal. My examination was mostly normal too, except for some sounds in your chest from bronchitis; and you're a bit depressed. I'd like you to take some anti-depressant tablets at night. They will take about a month to work fully. You won't get much benefit till near the end of the first week, though they will start to help you to sleep better straight away. I would like to see you again in a week.

RICHARD Could you give me something for this cold?

DOCTOR How does it affect you mainly?

RICHARD Oh. I just cough and cough and phlegm comes up. Makes me sick sometimes.

DOCTOR Yes. I'll give you some syrup to take 5 mL every four hours and I'd like to see you again in a week.

RICHARD Am I fit for work?

DOCTOR No. I'll give you a certificate for a week off.

RICHARD All right. I've been meaning to come and see you for ages, but I put it off, and put it off. Thank you.

## Interpersonal relations

### Non-verbal communication

The doctor adopted a friendly, welcoming approach with a smile, showing the patient into the surgery and inviting him to be seated. The signals both sent to each other were friendly, and almost immediately both were relaxed. They took to each other.

The patient seated himself on the chair farthest from the doctor.

### Rapport

Because he had never seen the patient before, the doctor saw rapport generation as the first essential. He paid close attention to what the patient said, listened carefully, making appropriate eye contact, and was careful to make appropriate verbal responses.

Rapport developed early in this case, but still the doctor was careful to reinforce at every opportunity. He showed a caring attitude by telling the patient to get dressed before he got cold.

Near the end of the interview he showed interest and concern by inviting the patient to return in a week, and met the patient's requests for 'something for his cold' and a work certificate.

### Confidence

Confidence in the doctor grew with rapport and was strengthened by his examination of the patient from head to toe. He was seen by the patient to be methodical and thorough.

### Agreement

Agreement was reached for the patient to take antidepressant tablets and cough syrup, and return in a week for review, and for the patient to remain off work for a week.

## General examination

| | |
|---|---|
| *Illness* | Obviously not in the best of good health, but not acutely ill. |
| *Intelligence* | Average or above. |
| *Co-operation* | Good, but with some reservations. |
| *Expression* | Sombre, rather unsmiling and immobile. |
| *Build and weight* | Slim to medium, but not wasted, and there was no oedema. |
| *Posture and movement* | Upright stance, gait normal, but he walked into the surgery perhaps a trifle slowly for a man of his 50 years and slim build. Later, while dressing and getting onto the couch, his movements were precise and well co-ordinated, but he was a bit slow. |
| *Temperature* | 37.0°C. |
| *Pulse* | 75 regular, normal volume and his artery was not perceptibly thickened or tortuous. |
| *Respiration* | Rate, depth and character normal. |
| *Blood pressure* | 160/110. |
| *Skin* | Sallow complexion, but no pallor, cyanosis or pigmentation; no rash, hair normal. |
| *Swellings* | Nil. |
| *Deformities* | Nil. |

## Regional examination

He was examined from head to toe according to the 'Clinical checklist' at the end of the book.

## Psychological state

The overall impression was of a middle-aged man of pleasant normal personality who was somewhat depressed. (See Appendix 3—'Clinical checklist'.)

## Summary of clinical evidence

The patient complained of tiredness, multiple pains, cough with sometimes yellow sputum, insomnia with early waking, anorexia and weight loss. His wife had died twelve months earlier suddenly and unexpectedly.

Examination revealed sombre expression, somewhat slow though precise movements and speech, blood pressure of 160/100, scattered rales in the lungs, in a thin but not wasted, middle-aged man. Urine examination was normal.

The overall impression was of a middle-aged man of pleasant, normal personality who was somewhat depressed.

Rapport was satisfactory, but confidence was not very firmly established.

## Diagnostic processes

### Pattern matching

The patient's sombre expression and somewhat slow speech and movements, insomnia with early morning waking, widespread pains, anorexia and weight loss matched closely with the doctor's mental image of depression.

Also the worrying cough, sometimes yellow sputum and scattered rales matched a pattern of chronic bronchitis.

### Hypothesis generation and testing

The doctor formed the hypothesis that the patient was depressed and this would be tested by giving antidepressant therapy.

The evidence on which to base a diagnosis of bacterial as opposed to viral bronchitis was considered inadequate at this consultation.

Similarly, the evidence of 160/100 blood pressure was considered inadequate to support a diagnosis of hypertension.

Additional evidence would be sought at the next review on both of these findings.

### Probability

From past experience, the doctor judged that the patient's symptoms and signs were due in part to depression.

The chest infection was thought to be evenly balanced as regards probability between bacterial and viral etiology.

Significant hypertension was considered improbable.

### Exclusion

*Cardiac ischaemia*

The patient described the pain in his chest as being simply part of his general series of aches and pains. He said, 'I've got a "cold", pain in my chest, pain in my back, pain in my head ...' In patients with acute ischaemic pain, it is usually the dominant feature of the clinical picture. The pains had been present for some time, as he said, 'I should have come to see you last year'. And it appeared they had no relation to exercise.

Again, the patient had very good peripheral circulation, with very easily palpable dorsalis pedes and posterior tibial vessels, and his radial vessels were soft with no hint of sclerosis. In addition, his urine was free of glucose so he was unlikely to be diabetic.

He smoked twenty cigarettes per day, which increased his susceptibility to coronary disease, and his blood pressure was 160/100, but he was a patient new to the doctor and could be expected to be a little anxious, which could easily raise his blood pressure by 10 mm.

A cardiac ischaemic cause for the aches in his chest was excluded on the characteristics of the pain, which the doctor judged to be simply a part of the series of bodily aches at multiple sites.

*Hypertension*

It is very common for a patient's blood pressure to rise in a consultation, especially with a doctor unknown to the patient, so the reading of 160/100 was not considered significant at this consultation. It would be checked as a routine at the next one.

*Asthma*

He gave no history of having been short of breath and gave no hint of it at examination, and he had no family history of asthma.

*Emphysema*

Again, there was no history of breathlessness and there was no evidence of emphysema at examination.

*Lung carcinoma and tuberculosis*

These could only be excluded by investigation, which would be arranged as soon as feasible.

### Provisional diagnosis

Chronic bronchitis and depression.

### Social diagnosis

A bereaved, lonely man of 50 years who had social strengths in his job and frequent contact with his daughter.

## Management plan

The patient was given amitriptyline tablets 25 mg to take three each night; this regime would take advantage of the sedative effect. The patient was asked to check the colour of his sputum, and given some linctus pholcodine to take in the ensuing week. He was invited to return in a week and to make an appointment on the way out.

The duration of this consultation was twenty minutes.

## Discussion

When the doctor studied the record, two points attracted his notice: the record extended over seven years, though with very infrequent attendance, and the patient had not formed a relationship with any individual doctor; it seemed he kept his distance from doctors.

Interview technique is always important, and so it was with this consultation. The doctor started by asking a very open question, 'How are you going?' because he didn't want the patient's response to be coloured by the question.

The patient did just what patients very often do, and expressed concern about a large number of symptoms presented in a rather jumbled way. It was an 'unorganised' story, typical of a new complaint which had not previously been subject to the clinical process.

The doctor focused attention on the 'cold', perceiving, largely from non-verbal signals, that it was the patient's main concern. He employed the technique of repeating what the patient had said, 'You've got a cold?' to avoid 'leading' the patient's response. He also did it because the patient had a strong accent and he wanted to check his comprehension of what had been said. The patient revealed that the 'cold' was really worrying him a good deal, and had been present for 'ages'.

At this point the doctor changed his technique from very 'open' questions to rather more focused ones, 'What sort of cold?', designed to permit the patient to describe his symptoms in his own words. The patient responded by saying that he was coughing up phlegm every morning when he woke up.

But 'phlegm' was not sufficiently specific for the doctor, who wanted to know exactly the character of the sputum. So he asked a series of focused or 'closed' questions, almost amounting to cross-examination, until he was satisfied about the reliability of the information. He judged it to be of considerable importance.

Here, the doctor was applying his facility for critical examination of evidence. He needed to be as certain as possible about the reliability of the patient's account of the sputum colour. So he pursued the matter till he was satisfied about its accuracy.

The doctor continued the interview, asking a series of 'open' and 'closed' questions about sleep, gastrointestinal function, body weight changes and the patient's work.

Then the doctor asked an 'open' question about the wife's death, having deliberately left it till later in the interview when he felt some rapport had been achieved. This was obviously an emotionally charged subject for the patient, and the doctor simply listened to the response, allowing the patient plenty of time to express himself. He also added some neutral comment from his own recollection of the event.

There were many questions the doctor did not ask, mainly about symptoms which might have been present. These included shortness of breath, swelling of ankles, palpitations, or CNS symptoms such as faints, or fits, or many others listed in the 'Clinical checklist'.

He also did not ask about smoking, because at this stage he judged it better to concentrate on building an effective clinical relationship. Questions and advice about smoking were judged better left till rapport and confidence were more firmly established.

Instead, the doctor relied on listening carefully, asking 'open' questions to encourage the patient to detail his symptoms and paying close attention to everything the patient said. He also relied heavily on non-verbal communication and general examination to guide him as to what questions to ask.

During the regional examination, the doctor exercised discrimination in each region and omitted modes of examination that he judged would not be of value or acceptable to the patient. This kind of discrimination is one of the skills that must be acquired in general practice.

As examples, one could cite vocal resonance and vocal fremitus in chest examination, and in the abdomen percussion, and auscultation, and rectal examination. These are all important modes of examination in the practice of which the general practitioner must be skilled. But the doctor must make decisions in each case as to what is appropriate.

The decision to do full examination from head to toe in this patient was based on data from the history, non-verbal signals and data from general examination. It also depended on the duration of his symptoms, the fact that he was a new patient to the doctor concerned, his age, and the all-embracing nature of his symptoms. This last virtually dictated that he must be examined comprehensively, as his whole body felt 'ill'. The patient's expectations would not have been met with less.

The doctor perceived a degree of resistance by the patient to his diagnosis of 'depression', which is 'psychological', and viewed as 'weakness' by many people. So it was with this patient. Yet the doctor decided to push on with it because of the benefit which could accrue to the patient. The doctor judged rapport to be strong enough to counter the patient's resistance.

Another approach to depression would have been to refer the patient to a clinical psychologist for non-drug treatment by counselling and psychotherapy. The doctor did not seriously consider this as the patient would have almost certainly rejected it and may have felt that the doctor wanted to get rid of him if he had been referred at first contact.

The doctor considered whether to give antibiotic therapy immediately for the bronchitis or wait a week. He decided on the latter, both because of the weakness of the evidence for bacterial etiology and most importantly because he judged the patient would not welcome many tablets all at once.

Why did this patient come now? He had been putting it off for a long time according to his own account. Perhaps depression could make him slow to seek help? There was a clue in the interview when he said, 'My daughter was worrying about me last night. When I'm asleep I jump.' Perhaps the daughter's influence tipped the scale?

* * *

Clinical method was applied in full because of the all-embracing nature of the symptoms, which required a comprehensive approach if patient confidence were to be adequate, and the doctor needed a full range of data to make a diagnosis.

## Richard—second consultation

*One week later*

### The record

There had been no contact since the previous week.

### Interview

DOCTOR How are you?

RICHARD Oh! I feel a bit better now.

DOCTOR Are you? You look a bit more lively than before.

RICHARD I'm getting a bit better sleep at night too.

DOCTOR They (antidepressants) do often work very well. I think they will work for you too because you've only had them for a week and you look much better. When that happens people do very well on them. You will get a lot more benefit in the weeks ahead. So you're sleeping better?

RICHARD Oh! Yes.

DOCTOR And you're moving better too.

RICHARD I've still got that 'phlegm' coming up with the cough.

DOCTOR What colour?

RICHARD Still yellow.

DOCTOR We'd better give you some antibiotic then. Are you getting any discharge from your nose?

RICHARD No.

DOCTOR Are you coughing very much?

RICHARD No, not very much; mainly in the morning.

DOCTOR Have you had a chest X-ray?

RICHARD Yes, last year.

DOCTOR We don't have a record of it here.

RICHARD Probably it was with another doctor. It was through work I think.

DOCTOR I'll just have another listen to your chest if I may.

RICHARD Yes.

*(There followed a pause while the doctor examined the patient's chest again.)*

DOCTOR I think I'll give you some antibiotic tablets to take one four times a day before meals and at night, and I think you should get your chest X-rayed again. I would like you to come back and see me again next week. Have you ever thought about stopping smoking?

RICHARD I've thought about it.

| | |
|---|---|
| DOCTOR | Well, we'll get your chest X-rayed again. |
| RICHARD | Yes, all right. What about work? When should I go back? |
| DOCTOR | When you feel well enough. I'll give you another week if you like? |
| RICHARD | Oh, I think I'll just have another couple of days, thanks. Then I'll be all right. |
| DOCTOR | Fine. I'll write that for you, but do come and see me again next week. You do look and sound very much better, but I would like to check you again. |
| RICHARD | Yes. |

## Interpersonal relations

### Non-verbal communication

The patient walked in more quickly and had a suggestion of a smile; he was certainly sending friendly signals to the doctor. The doctor reciprocated. When asked if he had ever thought of stopping smoking, he signalled a certain rigidity of attitude.

He still chose the distant chair.

### Rapport

Rapport appeared on a firm basis, yet the doctor continued to work on it by paying close attention, showing interest and concern, and responding appropriately.

### Confidence

Confidence was reinforced by examining the patient's chest again, arranging a chest X-ray and immediately agreeing to give antibiotic.

### Agreement

It was agreed to give antibiotic therapy for his chest condition, to continue with the antidepressants, to X-ray his chest again, and to stay off work for two more days and come back for review in another week.

## General examination

| | |
|---|---|
| *Illness* | He looked better. |
| *Intelligence* | Alert. |
| *Co-operation* | Good. |
| *Expression* | Cheerful, with some hint of a smile and less immobile. |
| *Build and weight* | Same. |
| *Temperature, pulse and respiration* | All normal. |
| *Blood pressure* | 150/90. |
| *Skin, swellings, deformities* | Findings the same. |

## Regional examination

The chest findings were the same.

## Summary of clinical evidence

Most of the symptoms of which he had complained at his first visit no longer got a mention. The only ones which did were his 'cold', cough and sputum. He also mentioned sleep, but only to say, quite spontaneously, he was 'getting a bit better sleep at night'.

Examination showed him to be more alert, speaking in less of a monotone, with less sombre expression, and a brief smile was apparent at one or two points in the interview. His physical movements were somewhat quicker. His blood pressure was down to normal limits, and his chest examination showed no change. Rapport and confidence were growing.

## Diagnostic processes

### Pattern matching

The pattern presented had undergone considerable modification, with lessening or disappearance of most of the symptoms and signs of depression.

Cough was the same, and the sputum was still yellow, which now presented a more definite pattern of bacterial infection superimposed on chronic bronchitis.

### Hypothesis generation and testing

The marked lessening of the symptoms and signs of depression following antidepressant therapy tended strongly to confirm the hypothesis of depression.

Bacterial chest infection tended to be confirmed by the patient's report of 'still yellow' sputum.

**Probability**

The likelihood of depression being a significant component in the original clinical state was greatly increased by the changes following anti-depressant therapy.

In view of the report of 'still yellow' sputum, it was likely that bacterial infection was at least in part responsible.

**Exclusion**

The disappearance of the pain in the chest, along with the other similar aches in other parts of the body and the now normal blood pressure, coupled with the enhanced clinical state, tended strongly to exclude cardiac ischaemia.

Chest X-ray certainly, and culture of sputum and sputum cytology possibly, would be needed, as in the doctor's judgment lung carcinoma had to be excluded; exclusion was required by the patient's age and smoking habits.

Tuberculosis also had to be excluded.

**Provisional diagnosis**

Depression and bacterial infection superimposed on chronic bronchitis.

## Management plan

The patient was to continue his antidepressant therapy unchanged and in addition take phen-oxymethylpenicillin tablets 250 mg four times daily an hour before meals and at night, and get a chest X-ray. In addition, the patient was to be reviewed again after one week.

The duration of this consultation was eight minutes.

## Discussion

At this review consultation, the doctor's aims were to detect changes in the patient's clinical state, to reinforce the relationship, to monitor treatment and to arrange further investigations.

In order to fulfil these requirements, it was necessary to again take a history and re-examine the patient. Regional examination was considerably curtailed, but general examination was repeated in its entirety because the findings were so important in assessing changes.

General examination showed him to be less ill, he was more cheerful in his expression, smiling a little several times, and these changes, though slight, indicated to the doctor that the depression was beginning to lift. Much greater improvement could be expected in the coming weeks.

As it turned out, investigations, except for chest X-ray, were postponed; the doctor sensed a need to 'hasten slowly' with this patient. He did not relish the 'sick role' and had put off coming to the doctor for a long time. He wanted only two more days off work and rejected the proffered extra week.

He was not impressed with the diagnosis of 'depression' and only half-accepted, half-rejected it. He saw his troubles as physical, and in his chest, and of course was partly right in this. The doctor also understood him as a person who would not accept a great many tablets at once, and so had delayed antibiotic therapy in order to keep the medication to a minimum. Now he had improved somewhat, and as confidence had strengthened, he was prepared to accept more therapy.

In respect of smoking, the non-verbal communication the doctor received associated with the answer, 'I've thought about it', indicated clearly that he had indeed thought about it and had made a decision.

The same kind of considerations applied to investigations. As mentioned previously, the doctor sensed the need to 'hasten slowly' with this patient. The relationship with the patient was of central importance in management.

**Outcome**

The chest X-ray was reported as showing early emphysema, but was otherwise normal.

He attended five times in this illness, and his physical and psychological state are well described below in the General Examination at his last attendance.

| | |
|---|---|
| *Illness* | He looked well. |
| *Intelligence* | Good. |
| *Co-operation* | Qualified by a new-found air of independence. |
| *Expression* | Alert and cheerful. |
| *Build and weight* | Slim. |
| *Posture and movement* | Upright stance and walked in briskly and smiling. |
| *Temperature* | 37.0°C. |
| *Pulse* | 80 regular. |
| *Respiration* | Normal, quiet. |
| *Blood pressure* | 150/90. |
| *Skin* | The same. |

In reply to the doctor's question, he said he had stopped the antidepressant tablets as he didn't think he needed them again. The doctor had no option but to accept this decision, which came as no surprise because he had perceived from the beginning that the patient did not really accept the diagnosis of depression. The patient saw psychological illness as 'weakness' and that it was 'up to myself', as he expressed it, to stay well.

The doctor judged it unwise, and possibly counterproductive, to again urge him to continue the antidepressant or raise the subject of smoking.

Yet the doctor had succeeded in establishing a relationship with the patient. This had endured through four weeks and five consultations, whereas previously the patient had no record of continuity with any doctor. Non-verbal communication on parting assured the doctor that rapport was alive and well.

The doctor reflected that free from his chest infection, with the support of his daughter, and the additional advantage of an established satisfactory work situation with its social contacts, there was a good chance he would remain well.

⋆ ⋆ ⋆

The whole gamut of clinical method was utilised: history taking and interview techniques, relationship formation, general and regional examination, assessment of psychological state, use of diagnostic processes and development of a management plan, which was monitored and modified according to early outcomes.

## Louis—continuing care consultation

This consultation is an isolated example of episodic care occurring in the context of a continuing care relationship.

### The record

Louis was aged 56 years and a regular patient for five years. In this period he had been treated for hypertension, with levels varying between a peak of 205/140 and mostly nearly normal levels of 160/100. There was a note that he omitted to take his tablets on occasions. He also had osteoarthritis of his knees, obesity and an alcohol problem. He smoked eight to ten cigarettes per day.

The family record showed his wife to be 48 years of age and to suffer from a long-standing depressive illness. One son, aged 16 years, was recorded as having a 'mild behaviour problem'. A second son, aged 15 years, likewise was recorded as having a 'mild behaviour problem'. There was no other information.

The patient had been an unskilled labourer until retrenched twelve months previously, and he was still unemployed. The family owned their home.

## Interview

DOCTOR How are you going?

LOUIS Ah, not much good, doctor. For two or three days my head has been whizzing round.

DOCTOR Going round?

LOUIS Going round: I drink a bit of wine, about a litre a day, and I don't do anything, but it still goes round.

DOCTOR When you look quickly?

LOUIS Look quickly?

DOCTOR When you move your head quickly?

LOUIS Yes. That's it.

DOCTOR Is there any noise or buzzing in your ears, or feeling like vomiting?

LOUIS No.

DOCTOR Well, let's take your pressure.

LOUIS I don't know; maybe it's a bit high.
DOCTOR That dizziness is not usually from pressure.
LOUIS No?
DOCTOR No. It's from the balance mechanism just behind your ear.
LOUIS Yeah?
DOCTOR Yes, but I'll take your pressure. (*which he did, along with the rest of the examination*) It's all right; it's not up.
LOUIS Well, what causes my headache?
DOCTOR How long have you had it?
LOUIS Oh, a month or a month and a half. But I didn't come, because I kept hoping it would go by itself. And yesterday the dizziness came and I was scared to drive the car.
DOCTOR What time of day does it happen?
LOUIS Anytime.
DOCTOR Well, I'll give you some tablets to try. Take one twice a day and come and see me next week.
LOUIS When? Which day?
DOCTOR Monday. The same day. Get these tablets and take one before breakfast and one before your evening meal, and take your blood pressure tablets the same as usual. Maybe you are drinking a bit too much wine. How much do you drink?
LOUIS About a litre a day.
DOCTOR That's a fair bit; see if you can reduce it to half a litre a day.
LOUIS I'll try. I'll try all my best.
DOCTOR Well, come and see me next week.
LOUIS Yes; goodbye.
DOCTOR Goodbye.

## Interpersonal relations

### Non-verbal communication

He was anxious and upset, but glad to see the doctor he regularly attended; he had a big smile as he came in.

He chose the chair more distant from the doctor.

### Rapport

Good; but the doctor took care to preserve it by attending closely and responding appropriately.

### Confidence

Strong; built on previous contacts.

### Agreement

It was easily reached as the patient was happy to accept what the doctor suggested. The doctor suggested what he knew the patient would be happy to accept.

## General examination

| | |
|---|---|
| *Illness* | Not very ill, and in fact looked very much his usual self. |
| *Intelligence* | Average or below. |
| *Co-operation* | Only fair at the best. He complies with his tablet taking fairly well since the doctor made special efforts to make it extremely simple. Previously he had been a poor complier. He is quite unco-operative in weight control, smoking and wine drinking. |
| *Expression* | A bit worried looking. |
| *Build and weight* | Short, thick set and obese, but not grossly so, and he had no oedema. |
| *Posture and movement* | Upright and quite bustling as he came in, his gait not appearing to be affected by his dizziness. |
| *Temperature* | 37.0° C. |
| *Pulse* | 80 regular. |
| *Respiration* | A bit stertorous in his breathing from his bustling, but it soon settled to quiet normal when he had been sitting for a few moments. |
| *Blood pressure* | 150/100. |

| | |
|---|---|
| *Skin* | Normal sallow complexion with no cyanosis, jaundice or abnormal pigmentation; no rash and hair distribution was normal. |
| *Swellings* | Nil. |
| *Deformities* | Nil. |

The doctor decided on the basis of history, relationship and general examination findings to limit regional examination to head and neck. The results are summarised.

## Summary of clinical evidence

Onset of headache six weeks previously, and dizziness two days previously, in a patient who was otherwise in his usual state of health. He had no tinnitus, nausea or vomiting.

Examination revealed him to be in his normal state with hypertension of 150/100, and head movements were found to bring on, and aggravate, the dizziness.

His gait and other voluntary movements were normal.

## Diagnostic processes

### Pattern matching

Headache unchanged over six weeks presents a pattern consistent with anxiety.

The pattern of dizziness related to head movements in the absence of other abnormal neurological symptoms and signs, apart from the headache, matched closely with the doctor's mental image of labyrinthitis.

The doctor had a clear mental image of the patient from past presentations, and the only differences were the dizziness and headache.

### Hypothesis generation and testing

In view of the features in the history suggestive of family malfunction in the shape of the wife's long-standing depression and the boys' behaviour problems, the doctor formed the hypothesis that the headache, unchanged over six weeks, was due to anxiety; this was not susceptible to testing.

The doctor formed the hypothesis that the dizziness was due to labyrinthitis and this would be tested by review after a week on medication, and investigation if resolution did not occur rapidly.

### Probability

The most likely cause of the dizziness was labyrinthitis; and of the headache, tension.

### Exclusion

*Migraine*

The headache had been continuous over six weeks, had not been associated with eye symptoms or nausea or vomiting, and migraine was excluded on these features.

*Menière's disease or syndrome*

As a cause of the dizziness this was unlikely, as it was unaccompanied by deafness or tinnitus, but it could not be excluded on clinical grounds. If this were an early case of Menière's syndrome, other symptoms would make their appearance with the lapse of time.

*Acoustic neuroma*

Deafness and tinnitus are the usual early symptoms and vertigo a much less prominent feature, and this condition was considered unlikely but could not be excluded. Review was necessary to monitor progress and referral would be necessary if there were not early improvement.

*Cerebral tumour*

The headache in brain tumour is more severe and tends to increase in severity. This patient had had headache for six weeks, but it had not been severe enough for him to come to the doctor, and when he did come it was for the dizziness, not the headache. It was considered unlikely on these grounds, but investigation would be needed to exclude it if it persisted.

*Transient ischaemic attack*

Dizziness is a common symptom of vertebrobasilar ischaemia, but is usually associated with other symptoms such as diplopia, dysarthria and sensory disturbances, all of which were absent in this patient.

**Provisional diagnosis**

Labyrinthine disturbance and partially controlled hypertension.

**Social diagnosis**

The patient was unemployed because of retrenchment twelve months earlier and had very little prospect of getting a job.

The family owned their own home, but there was evidence of some possible family dysfunction in the sons' behaviour problems and the wife's depression.

## Management plan

Promethazine hydrochloride tablets 10 mg twice daily for one week. He should continue his antihypertensive therapy, which required that he take three tablets together in the morning only.

These were:

hydrochlorothiazide 50 mg
+ amiloride 5 mg compound tablet;
clonidine 150 mcg;
propranolol 40 mg.

It was hoped he would be able to comply with this regime. He was invited to return in one week.

The duration of this consultation was ten minutes.

**Outcome**

He returned after one week to report that he was much better and very pleased with the tablets, which also cured his headache.

## Discussion

The interview began as usual with an 'open' question from the doctor, 'How are you going?'. Louis came straight to the point and said, 'Not much good, my head keeps whizzing round'.

The doctor repeated the patient's phrase on an interrogatory note, inviting the patient to enlarge but not directing him, while expressing interest and concern.

The patient repeated his complaints and introduced his own theory that it might be due to the wine. He also said he had tried resting, 'I don't do anything, but it still goes round'. Alcohol is said to be a factor in some cases of 'toxic labyrinthitis', but in this case was unlikely because of the rapid improvement on the medication.

'When you look quickly?' said the doctor in an attempt to overcome a partial language barrier. 'Look quickly?' queried the patient. 'When you move your head quickly?' answered the doctor, thereby acknowledging that his attempt to overcome a language barrier had instead created one. 'Yes, that's it,' came a very convincing response.

'Well, let's take your pressure,' said the doctor. He wanted to take it as the patient was under treatment for hypertension, but also because he knew it would be in the patient's mind as a probable cause of the trouble. He wanted to fulfil the patient's expectations.

The doctor did the head and neck examination at this point, and chose to make no answer to the patient's query about the cause of the headache, continuing to focus instead on the dizziness. The outcome vindicated this decision.

The doctor repeated twice his advice about how to take the tablets, because he knew that very often patients do not remember much of what went on in a consultation. There had been problems before with tablet muddle with this patient, and the simplest possible regime had been devised.

The doctor had asked for all the tablets in the patient's possession to be brought to the surgery so that they could be gone through together with the patient and confusion avoided. It had been decided that the patient should take one tablet from each of three bottles all together in the morning. This had worked very well.

The doctor suggested a time when the patient should come back, thereby underlining his interest and concern for the patient's welfare; this reinforced rapport.

The social situation was a major determinant in the patient's state of health. He was only 56 years of age, but had been retrenched twelve months earlier due to a factory closure and had been unable to find another job, having only labouring skills. He had no chance of obtaining work in competition with young, fit men. It was likely that these circumstances were responsible in part for his non-compliance with advice about weight control, wine drinking and smoking.

It had been suggested to him previously that he might like to join a group of other people in similar situations who meet for social contact, but he had rejected this.

The doctor did suggest limitation of wine consumption to half a litre a day, mindful of the fact that Louis belonged to a group in the community who make their own wine, a custom that was deeply embedded in their way of life. He judged this might be an attainable goal.

The doctor said nothing about weight control or smoking, as these topics had been exhaustively considered in the past with no result, and the doctor judged it likely to be destructive of rapport to persist.

The strength in Louis's social situation lay in ownership of the family home, and in their involvement in a strong cultural group in the community.

As always, non-verbal communication was very important, but especially so in this interview because to a considerable extent it made up for the paucity of verbal communication due to language difficulty. It was a very important component in the doctor's decision to do only general examination and head and neck regional examination.

The non-verbal message the doctor received was that the patient was really feeling quite well but was troubled by the dizziness, yet not too seriously. He projected his normal basic cheerfulness of mood very convincingly as he walked in with his normal upright posture and quick, precise and bustling gait. Had the non-verbal signals projected a change in his basic mood, the doctor's clinical decision to restrict regional examination to head and neck may have been different; it may instead have been to do a full head-to-toe examination.

But observation of this patient's posture and movement was a sensitive test of neuro-musculo-skeletal integrity and quickly excluded many problems.

A new doctor in the practice would have had to conduct this consultation very differently. Much more time would have to be spent on history, relationship development and doing a full head-to-toe regional examination.

An obvious source for some of this patient's symptoms was the nuclear family, since his wife had persistent depression which had resisted therapy over several years, and both sons had mild behaviour problems. Enquiry into these matters did not lie within the patient's expectation.

The difficulties affecting this family are highly complex psycho-socioeconomic in nature, and the medical problems tend to be a by-product of these more central problems. Any really helpful intervention in the family's difficulties would require full co-operation of all members and must await a more opportune time. The family must ask for help.

★ ★ ★

Clinical method included history, relationship formation, general examination and regional examination was limited to head and neck. Diagnostic processes rested heavily on comparative pattern matching, probability and exclusion. Testing of the anxiety hypothesis was not feasible.

# 6
# Care of the elderly

The next three consultations illustrate some important aspects of care of elderly patients.

## Henry and Alice—continuing care consultation

### The record

Henry, aged 81 years, had been a regular patient for some ten years, but had not been seen for three months. In that time he had been briefly an inpatient at the nearest public hospital for treatment of a transitional cell carcinoma of the bladder, and this consultation was the first since he had been discharged. He also had mild hypertension and giddy turns. These giddy turns were of long standing and had been very well controlled by promethazine hydrochloride 10 mg twice daily.

The family record made no mention of parents, siblings or children.

His wife Alice, aged 79 years, had schizophrenia many years ago and had remained very well on thioridazine 100 mg nocte and benzhexol 2 mg tablets half a tablet twice daily. She also has a moderate degree of sensori-neural deafness and is subject to recurrent urinary tract infections which respond well to treatment.

They are an elderly couple who live together in their own home and are mutually dependent. They do not appear to have any family. They are visited about once a month on a semi-social basis by the community nurse to check that they are getting on all right. They always come in to consultations together and are obviously mutually supportive.

### Interview

DOCTOR Good morning.

BOTH Good morning, doctor.

DOCTOR Well, how are things with you, Henry?

HENRY Not too bad; here's a note for you from the hospital.

*(There followed a pause while the doctor scanned the letter.)*

DOCTOR They've put you on some new tablets, I see; two to take after breakfast and one three times a day.

HENRY Yes; they said my pressure was a bit up in hospital.

DOCTOR Well, we'd better take your pressure.

*(Again a pause while the doctor took his blood pressure.)*

Well, it's pretty good now. So you had better keep on with the tablets.

*(Now it was Alice's turn.)*

ALICE I'm going a bit deaf, doctor. I wondered if I could get a hearing test in the clinic here?

DOCTOR Yes you can, but you may have to wait a week or two for an appointment. I'll just check your ears for wax.

*(There followed a pause while the doctor looked in her ears with the auriscope.)*

DOCTOR No, there is no wax; you can make an appointment at the desk.

ALICE Well, that's good then.

DOCTOR Well, come and see me again when you have the need.

BOTH Yes, thank you, doctor. Goodbye.

DOCTOR Goodbye.

## Interpersonal relations

These are considered for both jointly.

### Non-verbal communication

They both came in with happy smiles and the doctor smiled in response; they were both obviously pleased to be seeing 'their own' doctor and he was pleased to see them. They sat next to each other on the two chairs.

Rapport and confidence were strong, built on ten years of good relations.

### Agreement

This was readily reached with Henry by the doctor simply following what had been suggested in hospital.

With Alice, the doctor acceded to a reasonable request.

## General examination

### Henry

He looked well, intelligence good and unimpaired, co-operation was excellent, his expression happy and content, and he was of muscular build with no oedema. His posture and movement were upright and sedate, and he was slow but precise in his gait and movements. Temperature was not taken, pulse was 80 regular, respiration normal and blood pressure 160/90. Skin was normal and there were no swellings or deformities.

### Alice

She looked well, intelligence normal, co-operation excellent and expression content. Build and weight were normal and unchanged, and posture and movement normal.

The doctor judged further examination unnecessary.

## Discussion

Henry is cared for jointly by his general practitioner and the nearest public hospital, where the staff check and treat his transitional cell carcinoma of the bladder every six or twelve months.

His doctor has seen him at home on two or three occasions early in the relationship when he has been afflicted by giddy turns. These have never been precisely diagnosed, but have been very well controlled by promethazine hydrochloride 10 mg tablets twice daily for at least the last eight years.

When he goes into hospital he sometimes has been put on antihypertensive therapy because his blood pressure reading in hospital tends to be 10 or 20 mm higher than at home, where it is usually in the region of 160/100; on this occasion it was 160/100. Usually this therapy has been allowed to lapse after a period at home because he says he feels better without it. In view of his age of 81 years, his doctor applauds his wisdom.

On this occasion the doctor simply reinforced the hospital's advice to avoid contradiction; it is important for advice to be consistent. The likely outcome was that the patient would take the initiative to stop the tablets when side effects became troublesome.

Alice, aged 79 years, has been on antipsychotic therapy for many years, and the doctor has several times sought specialist advice about stopping her therapy, as she has been in remission for so long. But the advice has always been to continue. She is very well and able to carry on a normal life with the support of her husband.

It is a mutually dependent, stable social situation, with each supporting the other. The community nurse looks in about once a month for a chat to see if they are all right, but to date there have been no serious problems.

The nurse's visit is preventive of anxiety as it gives the elderly couple an awareness, and confidence, that help is at hand whenever needed.

This brief consultation, one of a long series over the years, reinforced rapport and confidence; the doctor met their expectations.

* * *

The doctor limited clinical method to brief history, reinforcement of a good relationship, general examination, and diagnostic method was reduced to comparative pattern matching, which showed them to be in their normal good spirits and physical health.

## Morris—continuing care consultation

### The record

The doctor knew Morris well, having seen him regularly over the last two years. Morris was aged 64 years and his record showed he had osteoarthritis of his back, knees and hips, as well as 'degenerative changes' in lumbo-sacral spine on X-ray.

He also had hypertension treated with propranolol 40 mg twice daily, prazosin 1 mg tablets, two mane and one nocte, and hydrochlorothiazide 50 mg + amiloride 5 mg compound tablets one every morning. He had also been advised to reduce his salt intake.

There was also a note that he was intolerant of indomethacin, naproxen and ibuprofen.

The family record showed that his wife was aged 57 years and was well. She had had four children, two of whom had died of fibrocystic disease. There were two children living, but they were not patients of the practice and there was no information about them.

Morris had recently retired from work because of pain in his back and legs, and he and his wife lived in their own home. He was an invalid pensioner.

### Interview

DOCTOR How are you going?

MORRIS No good. These (*patting his knees*) are driving me up the wall.

DOCTOR How long have you had trouble this time? I know you have had trouble before.

MORRIS Yes; well, I mentioned it to you before . . .

DOCTOR And we didn't do anything about it.

MORRIS No. Well, I've been away up to Mildura. Gee! I've been in some trouble.

DOCTOR Have you?

MORRIS I enjoyed the trip; enjoyed everything. And what did I find I was doing?

DOCTOR What were you doing?

MORRIS Walking.

DOCTOR Ah yes; it's not good for your knees.

MORRIS Lots of things I would have liked to go and see, but I was required to stand, so I gave it away.

I was in trouble again coming home in the train.

I had a case, and you know the ramp you've got to walk up? I got four or five feet over the dip and I had to give it away. My wife had to carry it up then.

I can't move round on it. See that there? (*indicating the medial side of his knee*) When I turn it hurts.

It doesn't hurt except when I go to turn. Then it gives me a 'turn'.

DOCTOR Well there's no doubt you've got arthritis in both knees. What have we given you before? Let's have a look. (*The doctor checked back through the record*) You've had ibuprofen, indomethacin and naproxen. Which worked best?

MORRIS (*with a laugh*) None of them.

DOCTOR Well, the truth is you're going to have to rest. That's going to be the best thing for you. But we'll try some

| | |
|---|---|
| | sulindac. You've never had that. The other things haven't worked or they've upset your stomach. Take one tablet twice a day with food. |
| MORRIS | I need to be on the go all the time. You'll have to strap me down. |
| DOCTOR | No. You have to rest. You have to do it yourself. Your knees will repair themselves if you give them enough rest. Rest is the key to the problem. When they've healed up, you'll be able to stand and walk without pain, but you'll always have to ration how much standing and walking you do. |
| MORRIS | I'm all right in the car; no trouble. |
| DOCTOR | I'll also give you some painkillers as well as the sulindac in case you need them. I'd like to see you again in a week to see how you are getting on. |
| MORRIS | Could you write out a script for that elixir to clear this cough up? |
| DOCTOR | Yes; the medicine works all right, does it? |
| MORRIS | Yes |
| DOCTOR | Come and see me next week. |
| MORRIS | Right. |

## Interpersonal relations

Both were quite relaxed in each other's presence and the doctor felt little need to be concerned about rapport; Morris sat close. The doctor took a directive approach, and after a small show of disagreement, Morris accepted the advice.

## General examination

| | |
|---|---|
| *Illness* | Not well, but not very ill either; not so well as at last contact. |
| *Intelligence* | Average and unimpaired. |
| *Co-operation* | Very good. |
| *Expression* | Anxious, a bit depressed, tired looking, though he sought to conceal his feelings and tried to present a good front. |
| *Build and weight* | Stocky, with a slight tendency to obesity. |
| *Posture and movement* | Bent over and limping slightly as he came in. |
| *Temperature, pulse and respiration* | All normal. |
| *Blood pressure* | 180/80. |
| *Skin* | Normal. |
| *Swellings and deformities* | His knees were quite swollen over the condyles. |

## Summary of clinical evidence

He had experienced a recent increase in severe pain in his knees, related to walking and standing, sufficient to threaten his independence.

Examination revealed some swelling of knees, tenderness round the joint line and marked crepitus in both joints, together with some reduction in the range of flexion.

In addition, he was somewhat anxious and depressed and looked tired.

Past X-ray examinations had been reported as showing osteoarthritic changes in lumbo-sacral spine, hips and knees.

Rapport and confidence were strong.

## Diagnostic processes

### Pattern matching

The pattern of evidence matched closely with the doctor's mental image of an acute flare-up of osteoarthritis of the knees.

In addition, he looked less well generally than previously.

### Hypothesis generation and testing

The doctor formed the hypothesis that the pain was due to an acute osteoarthritis superimposed on a chronic arthritis, and this would be tested by giving anti-inflammatory therapy and rest, and review next week.

### Probability

It was very likely that the pain was due to an acute on chronic osteoarthritis.

### Exclusion

*Gout*

Serum uric acid estimation would be done at the next consultation if there were not substantial improvement, but the history and physical findings did not support a diagnosis of gout.

### Provisional diagnosis

Acute on chronic osteoarthritis of the knees.

### Social diagnosis

A 64-year-old invalid pensioner whose independence was threatened by an acute flare-up of osteoarthritis in his knees. He lived together with his wife in their own home. He had strong rapport and confidence in the doctor.

## Management plan

The first treatment priority was pain relief, and to this end the doctor prescribed paracetamol + codeine compound tablets to be taken two every four hours when needed. He also emphasised that rest from weight bearing and walking was essential. Sulindac 100 mg tablets two twice daily were also prescribed as an anti-inflammatory agent; elixir choline theophyllinate was repeated in response to the patient's request.

The patient was to be reviewed after a lapse of one week, and possibly serum uric acid estimation and another X-ray if there were not considerable improvement.

Longer term plans included teaching him to avoid wear and tear on his knees whenever possible, and perhaps persuading him to take regular exercise by riding a bike or swimming.

The duration of the consultation was fifteen minutes.

The outcome was very good pain relief after six weeks and he was able to resume most of his normal activities.

## Discussion

The diagnosis of osteoarthritis was firmly established on clinical and X-ray evidence in the past, and the only diagnostic question concerned the nature of the pathology responsible for this acute attack. There was no evidence in the record of gout, though the serum uric acid level had not been tested. This was probably because the clinical pattern was typical of osteoarthritis, and not at all suggestive of gout, and so it had not been considered necessary to exclude it.

Doctor–patient continuity was vital in this consultation; it permitted the doctor to use pattern matching in assessing the patient's clinical state in comparison with previous contacts, facilitated diagnosis, permitted adequate monitoring of drug therapy and reinforced the relationship with the patient.

As with a great many patients with arthritis, choice of drugs had become a problem. Many patients develop gastric intolerance to the commonly used anti-inflammatory agents. This had happened already in this patient, and so he was tried on sulindac. Usually a trial of one week is sufficient to judge whether a patient will benefit from a drug.

A feature worthy of note in this consultation is relevant to all health education. When told he must rest, the patient said, 'You'll have to strap me down', but the doctor rejected this and firmly placed the responsibility on the patient. He was told, 'You have to do it yourself'; patients are responsible for themselves.

★ ★ ★

Clinical method was limited to study of the record, taking recent past history, general examination, reinforcement of relationship and regional examination of his legs.

## Ann—emergency call

A request for a house call to a woman with chest pain was received in the middle of a surgery session.

The request was from the patient's daughter, who said. 'What should I do? Should I panic?'

The doctor, though finding this a rather bizarre approach, merely said, 'No. I will be there soon.'

The receptionist told the doctor as he was leaving that the patient was a visitor and there was no medical record at the practice.

The doctor found the house easily, and after some moments of delay at the front door waiting for his ring to be answered, was at the patient's bedside within fifteen minutes of the call being received.

The patient was an elderly woman of 73 years who was moving restlessly about the bed, crying out from time to time, apparently in response to pain.

The daughter, who appeared young middle-aged, impressed as being ineffectual. She radiated nervous uncertainty, obviously unable to provide emotional support to her mother. She disappeared shortly after the doctor arrived.

The doctor took a brief history from the patient. The pain was in her lower sternal and upper abdominal regions, and had come on about half an hour before while she was having a shower. It had persisted since, had not radiated, she had no cold and had not vomited. Bowel function and micturition had been normal that morning. She had been in her usual state of health before the onset of the pain.

## Interpersonal relations

### Non-verbal communication

The patient communicated extreme anxiety and agitation, and her daughter likewise.

Personal space was not a concern.

### Rapport

Little; the anxiety acted as a barrier.

### Confidence

Uncertain.

### Agreement

The doctor assumed a completely directive role, tacitly accepted by patient and daughter.

## General examination

| | |
|---|---|
| *Illness* | She appeared extremely anxious and in pain. |
| *Intelligence* | Alert and answered questions well. |
| *Co-operation* | She was difficult to persuade to keep still. |
| *Expression* | Very anxious and agitated. |
| *Build and weight* | Slim, small build with no oedema. |
| *Temperature* | 37.0°C. |
| *Pulse* | 90 regular with a good volume and the vessel wall was soft. |
| *Respiration* | Normal. |
| *Blood pressure* | 140/90. |
| *Skin* | Normal apart from slight pallor, hair was normal. |
| *Swellings/ deformities* | Nil. |

## Regional examination

### Head

Rapid inspection revealed normal findings, including movements and speech, apart from an anxious face.

### Neck

The JVP was not raised and the trachea was midline.

### Chest

Chest movements appeared normal and equal on both sides. The apex beat was in the 4th LICS within the mid-clavicular line and was normal. Heart and lung sounds were normal, and there were no murmurs or adventitial sounds or friction rub.

### Abdomen

Inspection showed a thin, symmetrical abdomen with no operation scars or other abnormal markings. Skin and hair were normal. Palpation at first appeared to reveal tenderness in the epigastrium, but on re-examination this was absent.

### Arms and legs
These appeared normal to rapid inspection.

## Summary of clinical evidence
The patient had onset of chest pain in the lower sternal region half an hour earlier, and the pain had persisted.

Physical findings were normal except for slight pallor, anxiety and restlessness. Temperature 37.0°C, pulse 90 regular with good volume, respiration normal and blood pressure 140/90.

There was a letter which the doctor opened addressed to the outpatient department of a country hospital, but rapid perusal revealed nothing relevant to the current problem.

## Diagnostic processes
### Pattern matching
The closest match the doctor was able to make was only with states of agitation, anxiety and upper abdominal-lower chest pain, which could arise from many pathological processes; certainly cardiac infarction was one of these.

### Hypothesis generation and testing
The doctor formed the hypothesis that the pain was due to cardiac ischaemia or infarction, and this would be tested by investigation in hospital.

### Probability
The probability in the doctor's judgment was that the pain was due to cardiac infarction.

### Exclusion
*Cardiac infarction*

The hypothesis that cardiac infarction was responsible for the patient's symptoms had to be tested, and possibly excluded, and this could only be by investigation in hospital.

*Pericarditis*

The onset of the pain was more rapid in this patient than in patients with pericarditis, which is much rarer in the author's experience. In any case, the condition could only be diagnosed by investigation in hospital. There was no friction rub, but this is not a constant finding and its absence could not exclude the diagnosis.

*Pneumothorax*

This was considered very unlikely because of the absence of shortness of breath, and the presence of normal chest signs, but the condition would have to await exclusion by X-ray in hospital.

*Pleurisy*

This was considered very unlikely because the pain was not influenced by respiration and there were no abnormal chest signs.

*Lung infarction*

There was no shortness of breath, the pain was not related to respiration and there were normal chest signs.

*Acute gastritis*

There were no gastrointestinal symptoms such as nausea or vomiting, and though there had been a complaint of tenderness on first abdominal palpation, this was not present when the patient was re-examined. Other abdominal examination findings were normal.

*Peptic ulcer*

This was not considered a possibility because of the above considerations applying to acute gastritis.

*Acute pancreatitis*

Abdominal examination was normal apart from transient tenderness in the epigastrium, and the patient was not shocked.

*Gall bladder colic*

There was no complaint of gastrointestinal symptoms, the distribution of the pain did not conform to that of gall bladder pain, and the pain was constant and not colicky in nature. Also, the patient was slim and abdominal examination was normal.

### Provisional diagnosis
Myocardial infarction.

### Social diagnosis

As the patient was a visitor, the doctor lacked knowledge of her past history and social situation, except that she was elderly and had a young middle-aged daughter who seemed unable to supply emotional support in a crisis.

## Management plan

The doctor rang the MICA ambulance and arranged for the patient to be transported to hospital.

The doctor administered 10 mg of morphine part intravenously, but due to the patient's agitated movements the vein was lost during administration.

The doctor reassured the patient that the condition was not dangerous, that the pain would soon ease and that the ambulance was coming to take her to hospital to make sure she would be all right.

He then sat down beside the bed to await the arrival of the ambulance and occupied himself writing details of the history and physical findings and medication in a letter to the casualty department of the nearest public hospital.

The ambulance arrived promptly; the doctor explained his view of the problem and gave his letter to the ambulance team and departed.

### Outcome

The patient was reported to have been admitted to hospital with a 'mild heart attack'.

The daughter expressed deep gratitude for the doctor's prompt attendance.

Later, a report from the hospital revealed that she had been diagnosed as suffering from an acute inferior myocardial infarction. The ECG revealed ST elevation in lead 2, 3, and AVF consistent with an acute inferior AMI. The chest X-ray revealed no increase in heart size and no evidence of heart failure. She had been admitted to the coronary care unit and was subsequently discharged well.

## Discussion

It was a very anxious situation that the doctor stepped into when he crossed the threshold of the home. Anxiety dominated all three members of the household—the patient, her daughter and a young sombre-faced teenager who remained in the background following behind the daughter; probably she was a granddaughter of the patient.

Anxiety distorted the behaviour of both patient, who couldn't keep still, and daughter, who was at a loss what to do and tended to run away from the source of the anxiety.

The daughter was unaccountably slow to admit the doctor to an urgent call; later, she disappeared and had to be sought for some minutes so she could show the doctor the whereabouts of the telephone in order to ring the ambulance.

Her behaviour was due to being placed suddenly and unexpectedly in an unfamiliar and frightening situation; she was quite different when she spoke to the doctor in the waiting room the next day. Then she presented a warm, friendly personality. Such was the influence of anxiety.

In this situation the doctor became completely directive and made all the decisions, without attempting to consult either patient or daughter except to tell them what he was about to do. This approach was non-verbally welcomed by both; they wanted the doctor to take charge.

This visit was an example of a selective clinical approach in which the doctor assessed his patient rapidly and comprehensively, perceived anxiety as a major problem and adopted an appropriate response.

The provisional diagnosis of cardiac infarction was based on hypothesis generation, which could only be tested by transfer to hospital for investigation. Probability also supported the hypothesis.

In making the decision to send the patient to hospital, the main determinants were the probability of cardiac infarction and the intense level of anxiety in both patient and daughter. Hospitalisation would permit adequate investigation and exclusion of the conditions listed. Anxiety precluded any thought of home care.

Occasionally, in general practice one sees patients who, from their history in retrospect, have almost certainly suffered a cardiac infarction and recovered without any treatment, except 'taking it easy' for a few days. For some reason they have opted to forgo the benefits of medical treatment and hospitalisation. One can only speculate as to why.

★ ★ ★

Clinical method was reduced to brief history of the presenting complaint, rapid general and regional examination, and relationship formation consisted of applying a directive approach and complying with the wishes of patient and daughter for hospitalisation.

# 7 Child–parent consultations

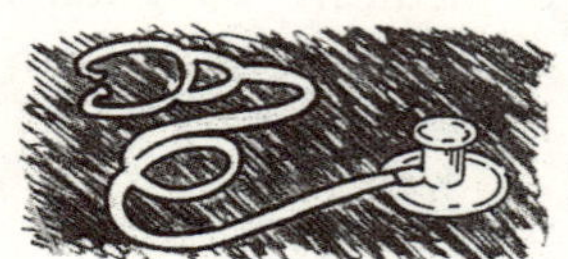

We now look at some points of importance in consultations with children and their parents.

### Relationships

Doctor, child and parent continually interact in a consultation, each influencing the behaviour of the others.

### The parents' influence

The parent-child relationship dominates the consultation. When the child has a close and loving relationship with the parents, there will usually be a marked absence of fear and the child is very easily examined. Competent parents prepare their child well for the contact with the doctor. In less happy circumstances, the child is obviously afraid and the parent may threaten the child with what the doctor will do if there is misbehaviour; there is then likely to be difficulty with the examination, calling for greater skill on the part of the doctor. These are the extremes; most fall in between.

### The doctor's influence

You, the doctor, influence the behaviour of parents and child by your approach. This approach should be friendly, attentive, relaxed, patient and caring. The parents will be affected through non-verbal communication; they will relax and start to grapple with the problem in concert with you.

You must establish a situation for the child which is reassuring, while not relating to the child except in the most fleeting way. Arrange for the child to be seated comfortably on the mother's or father's knee, if this hasn't already happened, or next to the parent and close to you at right angles and not separated by a desk.

Provided they have very close contact with a parent or someone else older and familiar, personal space is not a concern to young children, who come in without trepidation and sit right next to you. This is evident in the child consultations with Michael and George.

Occasionally, a parent accompanying a child attempts to sit the child on the chair next to you, with the result that the child obviously becomes fearful. Intervene and arrange for the child to be seated on the parent's knee. Such parental behaviour may raise doubts in your mind about the quality of the parenting.

It may be necessary if the child is investigative and active to reassure the parents that this behaviour is acceptable, while you both agree to keep a tolerant but watchful eye on the explorer, not intervening unless absolutely unavoidable. Such non-verbal behaviour on your part is very reassuring to the parents. They realise that you know how to handle small children.

### The doctor–child relationship

The doctor–child relationship is often, initially, entirely non-verbal and omits eye contact. You will strongly influence the child's behaviour by allowing the child time to become accustomed to the situation without the need to form any direct relationship with you.

You must be flexible and opportunistic in relating to the child, seizing opportunities as they present themselves, but withdrawing attention if the child shows any tendency to wilt. Spend a few minutes taking the history relaxedly from the parents, then make a very gradual and non-threatening approach. The relationship that you succeed in forming with the child and parents will determine the outcome of the consultation.

Relationship generation with the child and parents goes through the same series of processes of verbal and non-verbal communication, rapport generation, confidence development and agreement negotiation as in consultations with adults. The most important modifying factor is the relationship between the parent and child, which exerts a powerful influence on proceedings. Because it is of such crucial importance, parental confidence in you is considered in more detail.

### Parental confidence

Parental anxiety is at its most intense with illness in young children up to the age of about four or five years. Thus it is in dealing with this age group that you need to take most care to generate adequate parental confidence in your ability to manage the illness. Unless adequate confidence is achieved, the parents are unlikely to comply with management.

### Verbal confidence generation

Verbally, you generate confidence by responding appropriately to what the parent says, seeking more information or clarification on points as they arise, by taking a comprehensive history and displaying knowledge of the condition, and later in the interview you have an opportunity to impress by the way you give advice.

Some discussion should be entered into with the parents participating in the management decisions. Finally, there should be an expression of interest in seeing the patient again, and when review is essential, you should give very explicit instructions as to what the parents should do.

### Non-verbal confidence generation

You generate confidence by an attitude of caring, by close attention to what the parent says, by being relaxed and appearing so, and by displaying skill in handling children in this age group. Confidence is also generated by your appearing confident; confidence generates confidence.

Comprehensive head-to-toe examination of the child also helps to develop confidence in the parents. If they can see you taking time and care with their child, they are strongly reassured. In addition, success in getting the child's co-operation, and avoiding distress, helps a great deal.

It may be necessary in handling the child to begin very tentatively with the child on the parent's knee, and then possibly repeat some parts of the examination later on the couch when the child's co-operation has been secured. An initial successful consultation will make future consultations much easier. Finally, you should welcome, and invite by your attitude, parent participation in planning management of the illness.

## History taking

### Observer error?

Symptoms are reported mostly by the parent, which introduces the possibility of observer error. Therefore, the doctor needs to keep the critical faculty alert to assess the reliability of the data being collected. This may involve some cross-questioning of the parent, or child, if old enough, or other parent to verify some points.

As with adults, some symptoms are objective and some subjective, and the latter are not often expressed except very vaguely in young children, perhaps only as a feeling of general distress or feeling sore everywhere. Adults are able to articulate their subjective symptoms to a much greater extent.

Young sick children are very susceptible to suggestion, and questions as to whether they feel sore in the tummy, or elsewhere in specific situations, are very likely to produce affirmative answers of very questionable validity. Parents often engage in this type of activity in front of the doctor in an attempt to be helpful, but the end result may be only to cloud issues. More perceptive parents don't fall into this trap.

Objective symptoms are more reliably reported on and include cough, wheeze, vomiting, diarrhoea, discharging nose and ears, and the character of the discharge, fever, behaviour change in the level of spontaneous activity, appetite, fits or other loss of consciousness, falls, some types of pain, or inconsolable persistent crying.

It is necessary to obtain quantitative estimates about these symptoms. How many times has the child vomited today? How many times has the bowel worked today? Is the discharge watery, yellow or green? And how much of it has there been, and for how long?

When the parent says the child is not eating anything, the doctor may need to counter with a question such as, 'What has the child eaten today? At breakfast, mid-morning, lunch, afternoon or night?' Often the answers produced by this approach indicate quite a significant amount of food is being taken. The doctor pins the parent down to facts.

### Critical evaluation

This type of approach may need to be followed with all the symptoms related by the parent or it may not be needed at all. It depends on how precise an observer the parent is and how good he/she is at reporting. Taking a history via a parent necessarily entails an assessment of the parent. This assessment will be an important factor in designing a management plan for the illness later in the interview.

The adult history scheme outlined elsewhere in this book can be used, suitably modified, for consultation with children. As in adults, it is necessary to pay attention to present complaint, past history, family history and social history. In infants and young children who are ill, special attention needs to be given to the history of the mother's pregnancy, the birth and the early neonatal period.

In addition, if possible, the functioning of the family unit or household may need to be enquired into, as small children are totally dependent and may be severely affected by family dysfunction.

## Examination

Examination of a child is within the limits imposed by the child's co-operation, which in turn depends on the relationship with the parent and the relationship which you have been able to create with the child in the earlier parts of the interview. An effective relationship with the child is an essential pre-condition to examination. It is impossible to make reliable clinical observations of a desperately struggling small child. This may sound like a statement of the obvious, but it is surprising how often force is called into play in attempting to examine children.

### Take time

It is necessary to allow sufficient time for the child to settle into the consultation situation, and this time permits a full history to be taken from the parents. It also allows your relationship with the parents to be reinforced.

### Be flexible

Examination of a young child demands great flexibility in the order in which it is carried out and an opportunistic approach on your part. Thus, when the child opens his or her mouth early in the proceedings, you should seize the opportunity to shine a torch in and note the features of tongue, teeth, gums, lips, mucous membrane, pharynx, and movements of the lips, tongue and pharynx. This can be very rapid and obviates the unwelcome use of a spatula later in the examination.

If the child resists any part of the examination, it is usually better to go on with something else and come back later and try again to complete it. If this approach is adopted, restraining the child forcibly can almost always be avoided. Though young and immature, a small child is nonetheless an intelligent human being and should be approached as such by suitable technique.

### Play with the child

In securing co-operation, generally it is effective to use the child's capacity for curiosity and interest by allowing the child time to see, touch and feel examination instruments. This can be done in co-operation with the parent, who will nearly always participate in this play. The child can be shown your auriscope light, which can be shone on your own hand, then on the parent's hand and then on the child's. When this is permitted, very likely examination will be accepted. The same goes for your stethoscope bell or diaphragm, which of course should be warm. Looking, seeing, touching and feeling remove the threat of the unknown from the child patient.

## General examination

### Do it on every patient

General examination is done on every patient, begins as soon as the child enters the surgery and is carried on while relationship and history are being formed and recorded. It has at least equal importance with the same examination carried out in adults, and possibly more importance, because of the child's inability to verbalise symptoms. Non-verbal communication assumes greater importance.

As in adult consultations, the general examination findings, data from the history and the quality of the relationship determine how much further examination must be done.

The general examination is largely carried out visually, and is non-invasive of the child's personal space, and therefore needs no co-operation. It is mostly done from a distance and without removing clothing, and because of these aspects lends itself particularly to child consultations. The same routine can be followed as in adults.

### Illness

How ill is the child? Activity levels and vitality are a good guide in preschool and primary school-age children. But in neonates the illness of the child is not nearly so obvious. You need to observe the child closely, clothed and unclothed, in the parent's arms and on the couch before coming to a decision. A firm judgment may not be possible till the end of full examination and depends on integrity of the vital functions, the level of functional development and the nature of any pathology. If there is still doubt, it is wise to refer the neonate to an experienced paediatrician.

### Intelligence

Does the child respond appropriately considering the age and stage of development? Is the child aware of his or her surroundings?

### Co-operation

As previously outlined, this very often reflects the quality of parenting and the preparation of the child by the parent for the expected events in the consultation. Generally, children who feel secure in a close, loving relationship with parents are very easy to examine and co-operate extremely well.

### Expression

Is the child's expression alert, lively and cheerful, or immobile, frightened and angry? Again, this is largely determined by the parents and previous experience by the child of consultations with the doctor. When a consultation has been successful with a child in the past and ended happily, this will be strongly reflected in future contacts.

### Build and weight

This is determined by the child's stage of development, whether in the chubby small child stage or in the stage of thin body, arms and legs of five to seven years. Is the child obese, taking into account the stage of development? Some parents equate childhood obesity with health, and thinness with illness. They should be told that obesity is never an advantage and the level of vitality and energy of the child a much better guide to health than body mass.

### Posture and movement

Precision of movement increases from the gross movements of the infant to a high degree of precision later in childhood. Individuals vary in their motor skills. You must observe the child's movements and judge from past experience whether he or she is within approximately normal limits. Observation of voluntary movement is a sensitive test of neuromuscular co-ordination, and any departure from normal should be investigated clinically.

The child's ability to dress and undress should be noted and whether there is independence. Some children at a very early age, maybe two years, exhibit a high degree of independence and competence in dressing, with the parent hovering ready to help but allowing the child to do everything. At other times, a child of five or six years of age may just sit inertly and wait to be undressed or dressed by the parent as though it were a doll. The usual experience is between these two extremes.

### Temperature

In early pathology a raised temperature may be the only objective clinical evidence of physical abnormality, and so proper recording of temperature is of great importance. It is best to check it yourself, regardless of whether someone else has already taken it or not. You have to make the decisions and they need to be based on reliable evidence.

### Pulse

Pulse should be checked for approximate rate, rhythm and character.

### Respiration

Note the rate, depth and character, especially the presence or absence of any wheeze or stridor.

### Blood pressure

Blood pressure is not usually recorded in children in general practice. On those uncommon occasions when it is recorded, an appropriately sized cuff is essential for small children if the record is to be accurate.

### Skin characters

These are more readily apparent when the child is undressed and the whole body surface available for inspection, but an initial assessment can be made of the skin of the face and other exposed parts and of the conjunctivae. Is there any evidence of anaemia, jaundice, cyanosis, pigmentation or rash, and is the hair distribution normal?

### Swellings and deformities

These will usually be drawn to the attention of the doctor by the parent in infants and young children, and judgment based on experience is necessary in deciding whether action is required. Minor abnormalities of the feet are commonly enquired about, especially intoeing, and most of these will resolve. When in doubt, refer.

## Regional examination

The same pattern of regional examination can be applied in children as in adults, with the difference that full examination is done more often in children in general practice and there is need for much flexibility in the order in which the different parts of the examination are carried out.

Full head-to-toe examination of children is more often carried out because it strongly tends to build parental confidence. Full examination provides you with a comprehensive body of clinical data and ensures that nothing of importance is missed.

### Age groups and technique

The technique of examination depends on the age and maturity of the child and the relationship the doctor has with both parent and child. There are four age groups which require differing techniques—infants up to 12 months, preschool children 1 to 5 years of age, primary school children 6 to 12 years of age, and adolescents.

### Infants

Neonatal patients are always examined on the couch fully undressed in warm conditions, preferably on a blanket. Older infants may be examined at least in part on the parent's knee or more relaxedly on the couch. Infants are more relaxed lying down and easier to examine.

### Preschool children

Preschool children of 1 to 5 years make up the great bulk of really difficult child consultations. They test all the doctor's skills. Relationships reign supreme in importance and all the techniques of non-threatening approach previously outlined are needed.

### Primary school children

Primary school children of 6 to 12 years make up the next group and are a delight, because it is so easy to work with them. If your approach is relaxed and friendly, they are relaxed and friendly too.

### Adolescents

The adolescent group would not take kindly to being included here because what they most object to is being regarded as children. If they are approached as responsible, intelligent adults, consultations with them are usually happy. (See 'Adolescents', on page 99.)

## Systematic regional examination

We now go on to a systematic consideration of regional examination and the application of the adult scheme to the child.

### Head

The state of the fontanelle, whether relaxed and pulsating, or bulging, should be noted. Symmetry of the face and equality of movements need to be carefully observed.

### Ears

The ears should be inspected including the eardrums; it should be noted, however, that few observers can be confident about the state of the eardrums in neonatal patients. Inflammation in this age group is usually apparent from the child's reactions to examination or the presence of discharge. In older infants, the drums are easily visible and inflammation evident to the observer. It may be the cause of inconsolable crying, or caused by crying.

### Eyes

The eyes should be examined according to the same scheme as used in adults. Neonatal patients start to fixate at about 6 weeks and can follow a light, though you may need to repeat the examination several times to get their attention. Do the cover test in older children and note the light reflex. If there is suspicion of squint, refer early.

### Mouth

Children at all ages are liable to be upset by spatulas being thrust into their mouths, and the use of a spatula can nearly always be avoided. When examining infants, have a torch ready in hand and press gently and persistently on the chin, and you'll almost always get a good view, though you may need to spend a few moments. When the child does open its mouth it may only be for an instant, and the observer must learn to note very rapidly all the features in the adult examination scheme. Older children can nearly always be persuaded by gentleness. If they are asked to breathe through the mouth, a good view is usually obtained of the pharynx.

### Neck

The same features are noted as in adults; in young infants the main difference is to note how much control the neck muscles exert over the head movements. Always check for neck stiffness.

### Chest

The rate, depth and character of respiration has already been noted in the general examination. Check your findings again and note whether there is wheeze or stridor present, and if not, whether breathing is quiet and normal.

Inspection and auscultation are the most important methods of examination of the chest in infants and young children. Note if the movements on both sides are equal and whether rib retraction is present.

You need to spend time auscultating the chest until you are confident of the consistency of your findings. If you hear what you think are fine creps in an area, carry on and listen in all areas and return several times to the affected area.

If you are operating under the eagle eye of the parent, which you almost certainly will be, and you think you hear a cardiac murmur, don't dwell on it or you may be obliged to make an entirely unnecessary referral. Any hint of a 'noise in the heart' will mean that most likely the parents will demand full specialist assessment, which is expensive and should be reserved for those definitely in need. It is better to repeat your observations briefly at successive consultations to confirm the presence or absence of a significant murmur before arousing anxiety in the parents.

### Abdomen

The adult scheme can be adapted to children and infants. It is necessary to have not only a relaxed patient, but also a relaxed parent, because you need his or her help. Usually it is best to ask the parent to stand at the head end of the couch and relate to the child while you do your examination.

As with adults, inspection and palpation are the most valuable modes of abdominal examination. In an infant or small child with abdominal pain, you are mostly concerned to exclude acute conditions requiring urgent surgery. To this end, it is most important to detect tenderness and distinguish guarding from rigidity.

Palpate the abdomen all over with warm, flat fingers, gently seeking to relax the musculature and detect areas of tenderness. If, despite your best efforts and taking adequate time, you cannot exclude rigidity by achieving deep palpation in all areas, you are wiser to refer the patient for observation and investigation.

Abdominal findings will, of course, be considered in conjunction with data from history, general examination and the level of parental confidence in you. It is essential to act on the side of safety. If the child is crying inconsolably, beware of facile reassurance of the parents. If you decide not to refer immediately, check your patient sooner rather than later.

In such a situation it is an advantage if you can obtain a specimen of urine for dip test and microscopy. Negative micro urine findings will be very reliable; positive ones less so and depend on the experience of the observer and the method of collection.

### Arms

Ask the parent to undress infants and young children so that you can inspect both arms together in a good light for any asymmetry or rash. If possible, gently put the joints through a full range of movement.

The parent will almost certainly have noticed if the child is favouring one arm, and it is a good idea to put a direct question as to whether he or she has noticed any difference. Otherwise, the examination can follow the adult pattern.

### Legs

Again, insist on the infant or young child being adequately undressed on the couch, and inspect both legs together with knees fully extended. Look for asymmetry and inequality of movement, and note skin features. Again, make use of the parent's capacity as an observer. Gently put the joints through a full range of movement and examine for Kernig's sign.

### Gland areas

Examine cervical, axillary and inguinal lymph glands, and palpate for enlargement of spleen and liver.

### Skin

Always check all over the child's skin for rash; if there is a rash, is it petechial or a blotchy colour?

## Management of ill young children

### Beware of rapidly progressive pathology

Pathology in young children can progress very rapidly, and so you need to operate on shorter review times than with adults. You may need to review an ill young child after four, six or eight hours, or next day; whatever your judgment dictates as a suitable interval, so long as you act on the side of safety.

### Review early and often

Parents will be happy for you to review a sick child often and much less happy with longer intervals. The telephone can be used to do some of the review. Tell the parents of a child you want to review to phone at a certain time and say to the receptionist that the doctor asked them to ring so that they get put through without delay. Or if you want a partner to do the review, tell the parents the name of the doctor to ask for. Also, of course, tell the partner and write it in the record.

### Make precise, definite arrangements

If the parents feel confident of having the child reviewed after an appropriate interval, they will usually accept the need to wait and see. Your review arrangements must be precise and definite. Don't say, 'If the child is no better, come back'; tell the parents exactly what to do and that you want to see the child again.

Review should involve redeployment of your history and examination routines, and also it provides an opportunity to reinforce a good relationship. If you have recorded some of your findings, such as temperature, pulse and respiratory rates, quantitatively, review after some hours can reveal significant changes. On occasions, you may need to re-examine an acutely ill child several times to monitor progress and make a confident diagnosis.

## Danger signals in young children

### Vomiting

In an ill child, vomiting is always a high priority, usually the first priority. You must institute a suitable management routine of fluids, and possibly an anti-emetic such as promethazine hydrochloride by injection in suitable cases. Very often it is more important to secure the cessation of vomiting and adequate hydration than to make a precise pathological diagnosis.

Hydration can often be achieved by suitable instruction of the parents in techniques of giving fluids, a little and often, and to abandon temporarily attempts to give medicine by mouth, which is almost certain to be regurgitated. Paracetamol suppositories can be useful in such a situation. These measures, combined with frequent review, are very often successful.

### Inconsolable crying

If a small child doesn't stop crying despite all the combined efforts and skills of the parents and doctor, it is better for the child to be observed and investigated in hospital. It is wise to refer when you find yourself in this situation.

### Acute abdominal pain

If a child has severe abdominal pain persisting over several hours, it should be regarded as having early acute appendicitis. Acute appendicitis in young children is relatively common, and general practitioners of some years of experience will remember examples of near disasters or actual disasters because of failure to diagnose this condition early enough.

Localising signs do not appear early, and so they are a quite unreliable way of monitoring management. Don't wait for localised tenderness in the right iliac fossa. A more reliable procedure is to chart the patient's temperature and pulse rate over a few hours, and if the pain persists and pulse rate increases, refer early. Rigidity is present for practical purposes when you cannot palpate the abdomen with relaxed muscles no matter how hard you and the parent try to get the patient relaxed.

You may need to stick to your guns on occasions in the interests of the patient. If your patient, whom you have monitored carefully over several hours, is sent home from hospital after your referral, you may need to back your own judgment and insist on sending the patient back again with suitable communication for review at the hospital. This has at times been necessary in the author's experience.

### Neck stiffness

You should refer if you are unable to exclude this.

**Petechial rash**

Bacterial septicaemias and meningitis have become markedly less common in general practice over the last fifteen to twenty years, but petechiae are still a danger signal. Such a patient should be referred.

**'Ill' child**

Any ill-looking, inert child in whom you cannot make a confident diagnosis is best referred early.

Illness in neonatal patients needs experience to detect, so if you are uncertain how ill the patient is, act on the side of safety and refer to someone experienced in the care of neonatal patients.

★ ★ ★

We now go on to consider how clinical method is applied to a series of child patients presenting with very different problems and in very different circumstances.

# 8
# Child cases

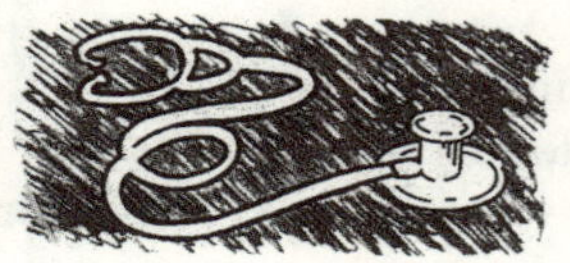

## Con

### The record

This revealed that the family were new to the centre, that Con's age was 8 months and that he had been seen by the duty sister as an acutely ill patient without an appointment. It was about 8 p.m. towards the end of a busy surgery session.

There was a note that the child had had all his immunisations to date, but no other information in the record.

Con was accompanied by the whole nuclear family, consisting of father aged 28 years, mother aged 25 years and brother Mark aged 3 years.

## Interview

*(The nature of the problem was obvious to the doctor as soon as the family walked in the door, because the baby's breathing was very noisy and of a familiar pattern.*

*After welcoming them and inviting them to be seated, with the patient on mother's knee close to him, the doctor said nothing, but merely listened from a distance to the baby's breathing for about a minute, or two.*

*All sat in silence for some time.)*

DOCTOR Noisy breathing!

FATHER A bad cough too.

DOCTOR Any vomiting or diarrhoea?

MOTHER Today, twice.
*(meaning two bowel actions)*

DOCTOR No vomiting?

MOTHER No.

DOCTOR He sounds as though he has a viral infection causing that—what we call respiratory syncytial infection. How old is he?

FATHER Eight months. He had some cough medicine from the chemist, but it didn't make any difference. It must be something going around.

DOCTOR It's always around. We see it every year.

FATHER He starts coughing at night.

MOTHER He's got a temperature.

DOCTOR Not much. They usually don't have any fever. We'll take it in a minute.

FATHER We took him to hospital four days ago because we thought he had croup, same as he did two months ago. The hospital doctor told us to keep him quiet and give him plenty to drink. We did that, but he's still not right.

DOCTOR Let's put him on the couch and have a look.
*(There followed a pause while the doctor went through his examination routine partly on the mother's knee and partly on the couch.)*
The most important thing is to give him plenty of fluid to drink, as the hospital doctor said. Give whatever he likes best to drink. It doesn't have to be milk. And don't worry about food if he doesn't want to eat. It won't

matter if he doesn't eat much for a day or two if he is drinking all right.

He has a viral chest infection and a red eardrum. I will give him some medicine to help his cough and make his ear better.

Have you got a medicine glass? (*The parents nodded their assent.*)

It's important to measure the medicine properly.

Give him 2.5 mL three times daily. You need to cuddle him a lot because crying makes his breathing worse. It's easier for him to breathe sitting up. His trouble sounds bad, but it's not as bad as it sounds. As long as he is drinking, he will be all right.

MOTHER Should we give him Panadol?

DOCTOR No. It won't help. He hasn't got a fever. I would like to see him in two days; on Monday night if you are worried, or before that if necessary, and you could see one of the other doctors.

FATHER Yes. Thank you.

## Interpersonal relations

### Non-verbal communication

This interview relied heavily on non-verbal communication, especially in its early stages when little was said. Instead, the doctor listened intently to the child's breathing and took care to appear to do so.

The rest of the family co-operated in this exercise and sat and listened too, and waited for the doctor to open verbal proceedings when he was ready. The parents communicated anxiety.

Throughout the consultation, the parents displayed excellent co-operation between themselves, each listening to what the other said and responding appropriately. They handled the older son with a high degree of parental competence and sensitivity. He spent his time exploring and asking questions in obvious attention-seeking in competition with the baby. They displayed a high degree of patience, sympathy and understanding, and handled him with a great deal of skill, so that the result was very little disruption of the proceedings.

This display communicated non-verbally to the doctor that the parents possessed a high level of competence and perception.

Personal space was of no apparent importance in this consultation, the mother sitting next to the doctor with the baby on her knee and her husband next to her. The small son spent his time roaming the surgery.

### Rapport

The doctor was at pains to cultivate rapport, as the parents were anxious and unknown to him. He attended closely and listened carefully, taking care to respond appropriately, and was rewarded by very satisfactory development of the relationship. It was almost all done non-verbally.

### Confidence

It was obvious to the doctor that generating confidence in the parents was going to be important, as they had already been to the hospital and the chemist without success before coming to the local doctor.

He sought to generate as much confidence as possible by examining the child comprehensively, demonstrating ability in handling young children, listening carefully to what the parents said and answering their queries, and displaying knowledge about the condition.

In addition, he reinforced what the hospital doctor had said and supplied some antibiotic, instead of simply advice or a placebo, in the knowledge that these had been tried and found unsuccessful by the parents.

He also invited the parents to come back, and explained how to do it, should they continue to be worried about the baby's condition.

### Agreement

This was tacit, the parents appearing to accept what the doctor advised and appearing satisfied.

## General examination

*Illness* Not very ill, though the breathing was obviously noisy.

| | |
|---|---|
| *Intelligence* | Appeared a normal, alert baby. |
| *Co-operation* | None. |
| *Expression* | Crying a large part of the consultation more or less loudly. |
| *Build* | Normal baby configuration for 8 months; not over or under weight. |
| *Posture and movement* | Normal for age. |
| *Temperature* | 37.0°C per axilla. |
| *Pulse* | Rapid. |
| *Respiration* | Very noisy, with both inspiratory and expiratory sounds; rate normal. |
| *Blood pressure* | Not taken. |
| *Skin* | No anaemia, cyanosis, jaundice or rash; pigmentation and hair appeared normal. |
| *Swellings* | Nil. |
| *Deformities* | Nil. |

## Regional examination

Due to the above findings and the parents' obvious anxiety, the doctor decided to do a full examination from head to toe. This was done partly on the mother's knee and partly lying on the couch.

However, as soon as the child was on the couch undressed down to napkin, he cried louder than ever. This permitted opportunistic inspection of lips, mucous membrane, teeth, tongue and pharynx without use of a spatula. The doctor seized this opportunity and also did rapid inspection of the whole body surface and palpated cervical lymph nodes, sought neck stiffness and palpated his abdomen briefly between yells.

There was much flexibility in the order of examination, the temperature being taken per axilla while clothed on the mother's knee, and the eardrums inspected.

Neck stiffness was also checked while on the mother's knee by getting him to follow a light travelling up his abdomen so that he voluntarily flexed his neck. His abdomen was again palpated for tenderness using the left hand with flat fingers, while the right rubbed his back as an aid to relaxation.

## Summary of clinical evidence

Illness of four or five days' duration characterised by noisy breathing in an 8-month-old baby, in the midst of an epidemic of acute viral infections.

He had been seen at hospital four days previously and given no treatment, apart from advice about fluid intake, and his condition had remained unchanged.

Examination revealed one red, swollen eardrum and loud scattered expiratory and inspiratory sounds in all areas of the chest, and he did not appear very ill.

The baby was a member of a well-functioning nuclear family.

## Diagnostic processes

### Pattern matching

The characteristic breathing in a baby of 8 months who did not look very ill, in winter, matched closely with the doctor's mental image of respiratory syncytial viral infection.

### Hypothesis generation and testing

The doctor formed the hypothesis that respiratory syncytial viral bronchiolitis was responsible for the chest condition and this could only be tested by observing the subsequent course of the illness.

A second hypothesis of bacterial otitis media could be tested by giving antibiotic therapy and review after several days.

### Probability

Probability strongly favoured the syncytial virus as the causative agent of the chest condition, and bacterial infection was considered the probable cause of the otitis media.

### Exclusion

*Asthma*

Asthma is uncommon in the first year; there had been no previous attacks, and the baby's pattern of breathing, though noisy, was not obstructed, there being no rib retraction, and there was no prolongation of expiration. Asthma could not be totally excluded on these grounds, but was very unlikely.

*Bacterial bronchitis*
This is very rare under the age of 2 years.

*Bronchopneumonia*
The child was afebrile, and most importantly was not very 'ill'. This is a valuable yardstick, but difficult to 'teach'; experience with children will rapidly give you confidence to make this assessment.

### Provisional diagnosis

Respiratory syncytial viral bronchiolitis and bacterial otitis media.

### Social diagnosis

An 8-month-old, not very ill baby supported by a well-functioning nuclear family.

## Management plan

The plan was to reassure anxious parents about a sick baby with a self-limiting condition which could be expected to run its course in two or three more days. The child had been seen at hospital and had also been given a cough syrup without benefit, and these circumstances together with a reddened eardrum persuaded the doctor to prescribe erythromycin antibiotic.

The most significant part of the management was to strongly reassure the parents as to the innocent nature of the illness. The doctor reinforced what had been said in hospital so that the parents received consistent advice. It was important that there should be no element of contradiction.

The other aspect of the management was to invite the parents to bring the child back again if they were seriously worried. They were told when to come back to see the same doctor, but that they could see another doctor at any time.

Duration of consultation was twenty-five minutes.

### Outcome

The family continued to be patients of the practice, but the baby was not seen again for this condition.

## Discussion

The doctor adopted an interview technique which relied less on the spoken word because the family did not have a very good command of English. This accounts to some extent for the stilted dialogue. The doctor stuck to short, direct questions and kept these to a minimum.

In fact, the doctor asked just four questions in the whole of the interview yet gained all the information he needed. He commenced with non-verbal communication, focusing attention on the baby's breathing and making it obvious that he was doing so. The family understood what he was doing, and waited and watched him. Then he made a verbal comment on the baby's breathing, simply saying, 'Noisy breathing!', instead of asking a question. 'Any vomiting or diarrhoea?' was the first question, followed up by 'No vomiting?', and later another question 'How old is he?'.

With these three questions, the doctor gained a full picture of the acute illness and some information about the past history of croup.

All the rest of the information was gained by attending closely, making appropriate eye contact with each speaker in turn, maintaining an interested expression and listening closely to all that was said. The father gave an informative history, without being led by questions, telling the doctor what had been said in hospital, and that they had tried cough syrup from the chemist on their own initiative. Thus words are not always necessary to establish effective communication.

This family non-verbally communicated two other very important pieces of information to the doctor; namely, that the parents were very competent, and that there were very good relations between the different members of the family. The examination of this child was done mostly to reassure the parents and get their confidence. It was a non-verbal communication to the parents that the doctor knew how to handle babies.

This examination demonstrates the flexibility that is needed in examining young children. It began on the mother's knee, was then transferred briefly to the couch, and then back to the mother again to complete it.

The doctor made a provisional diagnosis based on pattern matching perhaps thirty seconds after the consultation began. From then on, the doctor's main objective was to secure the confidence of the parents and their agreement to an appropriate management plan.

At the time, it seemed to the doctor that he had succeeded in these two aims, though he did not see the family again. Subsequent study of the record revealed that they had not returned to another doctor in the clinic for this complaint, and had continued to attend the clinic. So the assumption is made that the management plan objectives were met.

The diagnosis of respiratory syncytial viral bronchiolitis rested heavily on pattern matching and probability. The child's breathing pattern conformed closely to the doctor's mental image of the condition, of which he had seen many cases, and he was therefore very confident of the correctness of the diagnosis. The pattern of breathing, the fact that the child was not very ill, the age of the child, the duration of the illness and the season of the year all combined to strengthen the probable correctness of the diagnosis.

Hypothesis generation and testing were not of much value in this situation, as it was impossible to do any testing. Testing would only be possible by identifying the virus, if it were a viral illness, or by waiting for a number of days to observe whether the course of the illness conformed to that of respiratory syncytial bronchiolitis. The doctor had to decide how to manage this patient's illness there and then on the evidence available to him.

This highlights the overriding importance of clinical skill in general practice. The doctor must systematically collect evidence, critically evaluate it and subject it to a reliable diagnostic process. Thus are disasters avoided.

As regards the diagnosis of bacterial otitis media, which resulted in the prescription of erythromycin, there was no way of testing this hypothesis at the time; the doctor was obliged to act on the basis of probability. The parents had already had one medical contact, which resulted in fluids only being prescribed, and a chemist had supplied cough syrup, which had been ineffective. In the circumstances, it was very unlikely that their expectations would have been met without antibiotic therapy. Parental confidence had to be reinforced by treatment.

In devising the management plan, the doctor was aware that he was dealing with a well-functioning nuclear family with competent, caring parents. Had the parenting been of less quality, other options might have been considered, such as antibiotic by injection, early review the next morning, or even referral to hospital. As it was, he felt confident of the chosen plan.

* * *

Clinical method was modified by asking few questions, while relying heavily on non-verbal communication. The relationship with patient and parents was worked on carefully by paying close attention, displaying a caring attitude and making a full examination of the child. The parents' expectations were met and anxieties allayed by discussing the management with them as far as language allowed. And lastly, they were given specific instructions about what to do if they wanted the child seen again.

## Bill

### The record

Bill was 15 months old and the record showed that he had had a series of viral infections, but nothing else of note.

Family history showed that his mother was 27 years old and had a long history of renal disease, with many infections, and a small right kidney; she eventually had surgical treatment by re-implantation of ureters. She also had been in hospital for a serious lung infection that had never been precisely diagnosed. She had had three pregnancies with no complications, having two girls from her first marriage and subsequently a boy, the patient.

There were no records available for the first husband or the two girls from that marriage. Also, there was no information about her parents or siblings. The doctor had the impression that she may have been living with relatives on a temporary basis, but this was not enquired into.

## Interview

DOCTOR What's been happening?

MOTHER (*with child on knee*) Oh he had a bit of a temperature yesterday and a cough this morning. When he woke up, he had a rash all over his arms and legs. And he's got worse. His temperature is still high, he's pulling at his ears and he has got a cough. His cough is worse today.

DOCTOR When did he get sick? On Saturday? (*two days ago*)

MOTHER He had a cough Saturday morning.

DOCTOR Yes. No vomiting or diarrhoea?

MOTHER No.

DOCTOR Runny nose?

MOTHER No, not really.

DOCTOR Has he been drinking?

MOTHER Yes, but he's gone off his milk.

DOCTOR But he is drinking some fluid?

MOTHER Yes, cordial and water and things like that.

DOCTOR He's probably not eating much, I suppose?

MOTHER No.

DOCTOR How old is he?

MOTHER Fifteen months.

DOCTOR Well I'd better have a look at him. Come and sit next to me with him on your knee.

(*Then followed a pause while the doctor examined Bill, first sitting on his mother's lap, and at the doctor's suggestion unclothed on the couch. An attempt to collect a specimen of urine was unsuccessful.*)

He's pretty easy to get on with. (*a reference to the absence of tears or struggles*)

MOTHER So far.

DOCTOR (*having completed his examination*) So he has a viral infection causing the rash, the fever and the cough, and it's not all that serious. I think what you are doing is pretty good, giving him fluid and Panadol. I'd just keep on the same and let's see him again tomorrow. His ears and his chest are OK, and because it's a virus there's no point in giving him antibiotic.

MOTHER I thought it might have been measles.

DOCTOR Sometimes children do get a mild attack of measles even when they've had the injection, but they don't get very sick.

MOTHER My daughter got the measles when she was 5 months old before she had had the injection, and she got very sick.

DOCTOR Oh! Yes. Children do get very sick with measles if they haven't been immunised, but he has had his injection, so he won't get very sick.

I think you should keep on with just what you have been doing and let me check him again tomorrow.

Perhaps you could bring a specimen of urine with you tomorrow?

MOTHER OK. (*The child started crying at this point for no reason that was apparent to the doctor.*) It wouldn't have anything to do with him getting a new puppy would it?

DOCTOR No, nothing at all. You don't have to worry about that.

MOTHER I changed my soap powder last Saturday; that wouldn't have anything to do with it would it?

DOCTOR No, definitely not. It is caused by a viral infection. He will be quite all right. I would like to see him again tomorrow to see how he is going.

MOTHER All right. Goodbye.

DOCTOR Goodbye.

## Interpersonal relations

### Non-verbal communication

Neutral signals were received by the doctor, which he interpreted as indicating that not too much enquiry into the family background was wanted and that the interview should be confined to the presenting complaint. Wider discussion would not be welcome.

At first the mother chose to maintain her personal space and distance from the doctor by sitting on the chair farther away from him. However, she readily moved closer when requested to permit examination of the child. She also sat the child on her knee spontaneously instead of on the chair next to her.

### Rapport

Rapport was sufficient for immediate management of the presenting problem, but only just sufficient. The doctor worked to try and generate more rapport, paying close attention and taking care to appear concerned and careful in his approach to the child. This was successful with the child, but did not generate any more rapport with the mother.

### Confidence

The doctor felt that confidence on the part of the mother was at best tenuous, because of the failure to generate more rapport. He was still receiving neutral signals, though he had examined the child without any upset and demonstrated skill in child handling.

### Agreement

It was verbally agreed to review the child the next day, and to continue the same management of mainly fluids and Panadol. But the doctor felt this to be on an uncertain basis because of the neutral non-verbal communication which he continued to receive from the mother.

## General examination

This was done with the child on the mother's lap.

| | |
|---|---|
| *Illness* | Not severely ill. |
| *Intelligence* | Appeared normal. |
| *Co-operation* | Good; the doctor carefully studied his approach. |
| *Expression* | Neutral. |
| *Build and weight* | Normal for age. |
| *Posture and movement* | Normal for age. |
| *Temperature* | 37.8°C per axilla after three minutes. |
| *Pulse* | Rapid regular. |
| *Respiration* | Quiet normal. |
| *Blood pressure* | Not taken. |
| *Skin* | The skin showed a macular erythema on the face, limbs and trunk, not petechial in type. There was no pallor, cyanosis, jaundice or pigmentation. The hair was normal. |
| *Swellings* | Nil. |
| *Deformities* | Nil. |

## Regional examination

This part of the regional examination was also done on the mother's lap.

### Head

Scalp, hair, face and facial movements were normal to inspection.

The ears were examined by palpation of the pre-auricular region, gentle traction on the external ear and inspection of the drums, with the child sitting side-saddle with his head resting against mother; all findings were normal.

The nose was normal to inspection except for slight serous discharge. Patency was tested by gentle occlusion of each nostril in turn and observing that the child had a clear airway.

Mouth and pharynx, including lips, gums, teeth, tongue and palate, were normal to inspection, but as the child resisted wider opening of the mouth, the doctor left further examination till later.

The eyes were inspected and lids, lashes, periorbital tissues, conjunctivae and pupils were all normal.

### Neck

Inspection was normal and palpation of cervical lymph glands also normal. The doctor excluded neck stiffness by getting the child to focus on a light and follow it onto the upper sternal region.

### Abdomen

Palpation with the left hand through clothes revealed a relaxed abdomen with no tenderness, guarding or rigidity. The relaxation of the abdominal musculature was assisted by gentle rubbing of the child's back with the right hand at the same time as the abdomen was palpated with the left.

At this point the doctor asked the mother to undress the child on the couch, and this was accomplished without tears or struggles.

Further regional examination was done on the couch.

The whole body surface was inspected, confirming the features of the rash. The child was again shown the torch and gentle pressure made on his chin, and he opened his mouth wide momentarily, permitting rapid inspection of a normal pharynx and palate, and normal movement of the pharynx. The neck was flexed fully without resistance, confirming the absence of neck stiffness. Inspection of the chest showed normal configuration and equal movements with respiration. Auscultation of heart and lungs was normal.

The abdomen was re-examined by inspection and palpation, confirming the previous normal findings and the presence of the rash. Inguinal and axillary lymph nodes were normal.

## Summary of clinical evidence

There was a history of cough and fever for two or three days and a temperature of 37.8°C, and a macular rash on limbs and trunk.

Non-verbal communication from the mother indicated to the doctor that rapport and confidence were weak.

## Diagnostic processes

### Pattern matching

The pattern of evidence presented conformed closely to the doctor's mental image of an acute viral infection characterised by a rash.

### Hypothesis generation and testing

The hypothesis of viral infection could only be tested by monitoring the course of the illness and reviewing the patient.

### Probability

In the doctor's judgment, the probability was strong that this clinical pattern was due to viral infection.

### Exclusion

*Measles*

High fever, a florid rash on face and body, hacking cough, Koplik spots, in an obviously acutely ill child are features of a fully developed measles syndrome and were conspicuously absent in this child.

Modified measles syndrome in an immunised child could not be excluded.

*Rubella*

There was no adenopathy in this patient and this is the main reason for considering rubella unlikely, but again it could not be excluded.

*Acute bacterial infections*

Absence of any petechial rash, neck stiffness, high fever, severe illness and abnormal chest signs excluded septicaemia, bacterial meningitis and bronchopneumonia. Tonsillitis and scarlet fever were excluded by the normal findings on examining the throat, and the characteristics of the rash, and because the child was not very ill.

*Urinary tract infection*

This could be excluded by urine examination, but was rendered extremely unlikely by the clinical findings.

*Anaemia*
Anaemia or other haematological disorder could be excluded by blood investigations at next contact.

**Provisional diagnosis**
Viral infection with a macular rash.

**Provisional social diagnosis**
A frail 15-month-old child possibly suffering emotional deprivation with unknown family relationship support, and with a competent though perhaps unloving mother with whom the doctor had been unable to form a clinically effective relationship.

## Management plan

The plan was to continue rest and fluids as already instituted by the mother and review the child's condition next day, including examination of the urine and possibly a blood test. It was also decided to broach the subject of the mother's rubella immunity next day.

Duration of the consultation was seventeen minutes.

**Outcome**
The mother did not attend at the arranged appointment next day.

## Discussion

The doctor went to considerable pains to try and build rapport with the mother in this consultation, but was only partially successful, as judged from the non-verbal communication he was receiving from her at the end of the interview. It therefore came as no surprise to him when she failed to keep her appointment or let the clinic know she was not coming.

The object of trying to develop rapport with the parent is partly to encourage continuity between doctor and child patient, and partly to secure better compliance with advice; such had been the doctor's hope with this mother. However, it was not to be.

The reasons why rapport failed to develop in this case can only be speculated on. Perhaps it was due to the doctor's or patient's personality, or past experience by the patient, or some failure on the part of the doctor despite his best efforts.

Though it was the first contact with a doctor for this illness, the mother presented a very well-organised history. She was concise and factual, and spontaneously recounted almost all the things the doctor wanted to know. She had also done all the right things. Perhaps this derived from her wealth of past experience with medical consultations. She was an experienced patient.

The mother–child relationship impressed the doctor as not quite normal. She had done all the right things in caring for the child, giving fluid and Panadol, and bringing him for medical advice after two days. She had also provided him with a new puppy.

Yet she impressed the doctor as being unloving and distant with the child. She did not do the small mothering things that most mothers do, consisting of small attentions to the child throughout the interview, and didn't cuddle him. She was rather cold, distant and unemotional throughout, both with the doctor and her child. The doctor speculated whether her torrid personal past experience had rendered her thus. The child did not appear thriving to the doctor, and presented as perhaps a bit wan and listless, even allowing for the fact of the acute illness.

His physical state really did need further investigation. It was especially desirable to exclude urinary tract infection as well as anaemia or other haematological abnormality, but exclusion of life-threatening pathology was the main diagnostic concern at this consultation.

He started to cry for no apparent reason after all the examination was over, and the doctor thought it possible this could have been due to a degree of emotional deprivation. The failure of the mother to return prevented any further exploration of the relationship or pathology. Those most in need of counselling are often the hardest to persuade to undertake it.

* * *

Because of concern about the child, the doctor applied the full clinical method; there were no shortcuts.

## Michael—first consultation

### The record

Michael was 2 years old and had attended on four previous occasions with viral infections and otitis media. His immunisations were up to date. There was no other information about him. His mother was 26 years old and well, and his father was 25 years of age and well. The family was new in the area and no other member of the family had attended the clinic.

On this occasion he was brought by a young adolescent boy, aged about 13 or 14 years, whom the doctor at first wrongly assumed to be an elder brother. The relationship was never clarified.

### Interview

DOCTOR What's the matter?

FRIEND He's been complaining that his ears are sore.

DOCTOR Has he got a cold?

FRIEND Yes; I think he's got one.

DOCTOR Has he got a cough?

FRIEND He did have one a couple of weeks ago, but not now.

DOCTOR No vomiting or diarrhoea?

FRIEND No.

DOCTOR Nose not running?

FRIEND Yes.

DOCTOR And how long has he had that?

FRIEND Probably about a week or more, I'd say.

DOCTOR That long; and he's eating?

FRIEND Not much. He's got blood all over his nose all the time as soon as he gets a cold.

(*At this point the doctor went straight to the probable source of trouble and had a look in both of the child's ears with his auriscope, taking care to make a friendly approach to the child.*)

Yesterday some pus or something came out of this eye here.

DOCTOR Were his eyelids stuck together this morning?

FRIEND No.

DOCTOR Probably the pus was coming from the corner near his nose?

FRIEND Yes.

DOCTOR Well, that's an infection in his tear duct.

FRIEND When he gets a cold his nose bleeds often.

DOCTOR Which side?

FRIEND Both sides.

(*The doctor examined his nose, throat and ears again.*)

DOCTOR I'll give him some medicine, antibiotic, to take 5 mL twice a day and some pseudoephedrine syrup to take 5 mL four times a day. And I want to see him again to have another look at his eardrums even if he seems perfectly well next week. I'd like to see him again next Monday night.

FRIEND OK then; goodbye.

DOCTOR Goodbye.

## Interpersonal relations

### Non-verbal communication

The child, though only about 2 years of age, walked in confidently holding hands with the older boy accompanying him. The pair of them sat down quietly on two chairs next to the doctor and proceedings began without any difficulty. They were neither fearful nor overconfident. Personal space was not a problem as the young patient came and sat right next to the doctor.

In conformity with his usual practice, and to give the young child time to become accustomed to the situation, the doctor did no more than give him a fleeting glance at first; he directed attention to the older child, making eye contact with him.

### Rapport

This developed easily because of the unusually co-operative nature of the young patient, and was built up by the doctor carefully studying his approach.

Various rapport-generation techniques were put into operation. These included avoidance of early eye contact and gentle palpation of cervical glands with warm hands. Then the child was shown the torch, which the doctor shone on his own hand first, giving the child plenty of time to see it and appreciate it for a non-threatening object. Then it was shone on the hand of the older boy, who co-operated in this game and then on the young patient's hand. He permitted this to happen and did not pull his hand away. This signalled to the doctor that he was ready to permit more examination.

### Confidence

This developed successfully because the doctor had developed adequate rapport. In this situation with two such young persons, confidence almost entirely depended on rapport.

### Agreement

Agreement on the management regime proposed by the doctor was immediate. There were no difficulties.

## General examination

This showed the patient to be not seriously ill, intelligent, co-operative and alert, and of average build and weight for a 2-year-old. He walked and moved normally, and his temperature was 37.2°C per axilla after three minutes. His other general examination findings were normal.

## Summary of clinical evidence

The child had a history of a 'cold' over the last week, with discharging nose, nose bleeds, discharge from his eye and sore ears.

This child was not very ill, was alert and co-operative, with normal posture and movement, and normal temperature, pulse, respiration and skin characters.

Regional examination revealed bilateral red swollen eardrums, some obstruction to the nose and discharge from the left naso lacrimal papilla.

The family and social situation were unknown.

## Diagnostic processes

### Pattern matching

Sore ears, red bulging eardrums and a recent cold matched closely with the doctor's mental image of otitis media.

A cold for a week, accompanied by nose bleeds, discharge from the nose and purulent discharge from the lacrimal papilla, matched a pattern of sinusitis.

### Hypothesis generation and testing

On the above evidence and the purulent discharge from the naso lacrimal papilla, the doctor formed the hypothesis that the child had bacterial otitis media and sinusitis, and this would be tested by giving antibiotic therapy and review.

### Probability

The doctor judged the most likely diagnosis was bacterial otitis media and sinusitis; the likelihood was that the maxillary sinus was infected as well as the naso lacrimal duct. Frontal sinusitis is uncommon before the age of 3 years.

### Exclusion

*Nasal foreign body*

The child's nose was examined with a light, which permitted only inspection of the anterior nares. No foreign body was visible, but any further examination with instruments would require the presence and consent of a parent. Exclusion was not possible at this consultation.

*Chronic otitis media*

This could not be excluded at this consultation; re-examination at review would be necessary.

### Provisional diagnosis

Bilateral otitis media and sinusitis.

### Provisional social diagnosis

A 2-year-old child with unknown family relationship support.

## Management plan

The doctor prescribed phenoxymethylpenicillin 125 mg per 5 mL four times daily for five days and elixir pseudoephedrine 5 mL four times daily for two days. An appointment was made in a week in the evening because both parents worked, and the doctor wanted to meet at least one of them. Also, he wanted to review the child's general clinical condition, and check the state of the eardrums and nose.

Duration of consultation was ten minutes.

### Discussion

This interview was strongly influenced by the patient's age of 2 years, the absence of both parents, the fact that they were new patients to the doctor and the age of the teenager accompanying the patient.

In the circumstances, the doctor modified his technique considerably. He asked short, direct questions designed to provide maximum information about the child's recent and present physical state, while maintaining a cheerful and buoyant tone.

In fact, the child turned out to be exceptionally easy to manage for a 2-year-old, and the adolescent behaved with considerable maturity. Precise and definite answers were given, and he volunteered some useful information on his own initiative.

Had a parent been present, the approach would have been quite a lot different in that the doctor would also have been asking open-ended questions to get information about the parent and child–parent relationship.

Another reason for the limited questions was that the doctor felt it would be putting an unfair strain on a youngish adolescent to ask much about past history and quite inappropriate to launch into family or social history.

As always, important decisions flowed from the general examination findings. The most important observation was that the child was not very ill. Had the child been very ill, there would have been need to urgently contact the parents.

The absence of parents also caused some limitation of examination, as the doctor felt the child needed the support of a parent if there were to be full regional examination. Small children often find being undressed in the surgery threatening and fight against it. The doctor felt that full examination might put too much stress on the relationship, and as the child was not very ill, examination was reduced to the barest minimum.

The doctor took considerable care to cultivate favourable relations, using rapport-generation techniques with the child, and with the accompanying adolescent. In fact, it turned out to be an outstandingly successful consultation considering the age of the patient and other adverse factors. The doctor was favourably impressed by the two and suspected that it might reflect good quality parenting. It is usual to find children who have a very secure relationship with their parents easy to examine. He also suspected they were of good intelligence.

The doctor opted for oral treatment of the patient instead of an injection, which would have been invasive and required specific authority of the parents. In any case, the doctor would have avoided it if possible as injections seriously impair doctor–child patient relations.

## Michael—second consultation

### The record

The record showed he had not attended the clinic in the past week.

### Interview

DOCTOR How's he going?

MOTHER Pretty well; keeps talking about it.

DOCTOR Would you take his coat off? He seems fairly well to you, does he? Let's have a look in his ears; that one looks good and so does the other. And his nose seems quite clear too. (*to mother*) He has been taking his medicine for a week now and it has worked well, so it can be stopped. (*to the patient*) So we'll have to hope you don't get sore ears again.

MOTHER I used to get them myself when I was young.

DOCTOR Well, let's see him again if there is any more trouble.

## Interpersonal relations

### Non-verbal communication

This time there were two people sending signals and they were both relaxed and friendly. Mother and son walked in together much as had happened the week before, but then with a young adolescent boy instead of mother. Again there was the same relaxed confident atmosphere.

The doctor perceived that the signals between mother and son were similarly relaxed and friendly. Mother did the normal mothering things of sitting him on her knee and giving him a constant series of little attentions. He snuggled against her. She chose the chair next to the doctor; both were comfortable close to him.

### Rapport

This was easily established with the mother and son; there were no reservations.

### Confidence

This seemed to the doctor to be very good, despite mother and doctor being new to each other.

### Agreement

Agreement was easily reached as all that was involved was to stop the medicine and return if there were any future problems.

## Summary of clinical evidence

Generally, he looked very well and regional examination was normal, and he had a happy normal relationship with his mother.

### Diagnosis

Healthy child following resolution of bacterial otitis media and sinusitis.

## Management plan

The mother was invited to bring him back if there were any further trouble.

Duration of consultation was four minutes.

## Discussion

This consultation had been arranged by the doctor with the dual purpose of meeting one or other of the parents and establishing a relationship with a family new to the area, and the doctor wanted to check that the otitis media and sinusitis had completely resolved.

This consultation was notable for the ease and rapidity with which rapport developed. A favourable relationship was established immediately despite the brevity of the consultation, and the doctor felt confident that the family would become established patients. The best care depends on continuity. This was the doctor's object in seeking to establish a relationship with the parents.

It was essential for the doctor to check the child's ears to ensure resolution was complete, as there had already been several similar episodes.

★ ★ ★

The clinical method was abbreviated at the first consultation by not taking a full history from the young adolescent, and limiting regional examination to ear, nose and throat.

At the second consultation, clinical method was curtailed because of the obvious improvement in general examination findings. Regional examination was limited to ear, nose and throat. Relationship development with the mother was carried on largely non-verbally.

# George—first consultation

### The record

George was 3 years old, and ten months previously had had an operation for an undescended testicle.

Post-operatively the wound had gaped and there had been a series of visits for dressings.

Mother was aged 40 years, but there was no other information about her.

Father was aged 41 years, suffered from hypertension and had had an attack of ischaemic chest pain last year.

A brother, aged 19 years, had psittacosis last year and two years ago had suffered a head injury, which resulted in persistent headaches. He also had congenital nystagmus.

Another brother, aged 18 years, had had a knee injury.

The family live in their own home, supported by father, who has a responsible job, and mother, who is a full-time homemaker.

## Interview

(*George was accompanied by his 19-year-old brother.*)

DOCTOR Come in and have a seat. What's been happening to George?

BROTHER He's been complaining for a couple of months; all the time he gets 'pains' round the lower part of his stomach.

DOCTOR Aha! How old is he?

BROTHER Three years.

DOCTOR Is there anything you've noticed that seems to bring it on?

BROTHER Oh no, no. It was mainly this morning walking to kinder, and he reckons he keeps getting pain in his stomach. All the time he kept saying he had a pain in there somewhere. (*indicating the lower abdomen of his young brother sitting on the chair next to him*)

DOCTOR Yes; and it's been for several months?

BROTHER Yes. We just thought, you know, that we should get it checked.

DOCTOR Well, he might be worried about something. Quite often young children do get worried about things and it comes out as pain. They express their worry as pain in the tummy. He might be a bit nervous about going to kinder.

BROTHER He's had it since before he went to kinder.

DOCTOR Has he?

BROTHER Yes; mainly since he had his operation.

DOCTOR What was that for?

BROTHER Testicle, I think.

DOCTOR How long ago was that?

BROTHER I don't know; could be a year.

DOCTOR Last year! (*scrutinising the history*)

BROTHER He's had diarrhoea lately too.

DOCTOR How much today?

BROTHER Oh none today.

DOCTOR Yes; and no vomiting today?

BROTHER He kept saying he wanted to go to the toilet to do pooh; when he gets there, he says his bum is sore.

DOCTOR Yes, yes; and he passes water all right?

BROTHER Oh yeah; a bit too much.

DOCTOR Has he got any cough or cold?

BROTHER No.

DOCTOR Well, we'd better have a look at you, hadn't we? (*This was addressed to the patient, who had been sitting on his own chair next to the doctor and beside his big brother all through this exchange, saying nothing at all.*)

Can you pop this under your arm, George?

(*The doctor put a thermometer under his arm, getting him to wrap his other arm over the one with the thermometer to keep it snug, and making sure in the process that it was really in the skin fold, with no intervening clothes.*)

Let's have a look at your tongue?

(*The doctor felt for glands at the same time, and afterwards shone a torch on his own hand, then on George's, to which the patient submitted with interest, having a good look at it.*

*After this play, George opened his mouth wide when requested, providing a good view of his mouth and pharynx. The doctor made a rapid assessment of lips, mucous membrane, tongue, teeth, tonsils and palate, all of which were normal. Finally, he was persuaded to say 'Ah!' all without a spatula.*)

Sniff in!

(*George co-operated and allowed each nostril to be gently occluded while he sniffed in through the other. He was actively starting to co-operate.*

*Next, the doctor showed George his auriscope light, shone it on his own hand,*

*and then on George's, and then was permitted to shine it in George's ear. The patient willingly turned his head to permit the light to be shone in his other ear, so that the doctor obtained a clear, unhurried view of each eardrum.*

*The doctor noted that the patient had a rotational nystagmus affecting both eyes.)*

He's got wobbly eyes.

BROTHER Yes, same as me.

DOCTOR You've got them too?

BROTHER Yes, it's nystagmus.

(*At this point the child was very relaxed and permitted his abdomen to be gently but firmly palpated. The doctor was able without any struggling or opposition to determine very convincingly that there was no tenderness or rigidity. He succeeded in palpating deeply in all areas, assisted by giving the child a rub on the back at the same time with his non-palpating hand, which further assisted in relaxing the abdominal musculature.*

*The doctor then warmed his stethoscope diaphragm under the hot tap and lifted the child's clothes and listened to all areas of the chest, first taking care to let George look for several minutes at the diaphragm and feel it. Then it was rubbed on George's hand and then on his chest before finally listening. Auscultatory findings were then free of any extraneous sounds. This technique permitted a large measure of confidence in the reliability of the examination findings.*)

DOCTOR Can you come and lie on the bed? We've got a step here. Can you climb up there? I just want to feel your tummy. Climb up there and lie down for me.

(*George complied readily and was very easy to examine. The doctor made sure his hands were warm and handled the child gently. George now had all his clothes removed except for underpants, so that full inspection was possible from head to toe.*

*Respiratory movements were quickly noted, as was the child's relaxed attitude on the couch. The head was gently flexed, cervical glands palpated, nasal airway rechecked, and the child readily opened his mouth so that oral findings could be checked.*

*Eardrums were visualised again, and chest and heart auscultated and abdomen re-examined. Penis and scrotum were inspected, and testes and hernial orifices palpated.*

*His legs and arms were rapidly inspected, including movements. The joints were put through a full range of movement. George's movements as he got on and off the couch were noted to be deft and well co-ordinated.*)

I wonder if he could pass some urine for us?

(*George demurred, but was soon persuaded to try. The doctor supposed that most people perform better without spectators and that George could go into the next room, but it didn't work.*)

I can't find anything physically wrong with him. I think it's a worry type sore tummy. You know, kids often get symptoms and things wrong with them after they've been in hospital and had an operation: that's quite a worrying thing to happen to a small child. How long was he in?

BROTHER Oh, only a couple of days, but then just afterwards the stitches broke and it got infected, which caused a deal of trouble.

DOCTOR Well, what I think he needs is lots of love and cuddles. Could you get his mother to bring him up tomorrow and bring a specimen of urine?

BROTHER Yes.

DOCTOR I can't find anything wrong with him, but I would like to check him again tomorrow and talk to his mother. Make an appointment now because I would like to see him again.

Come and see us again tomorrow night?

(*This was said to George, who answered 'Yes' quite independently and without coaxing.*)

DOCTOR Goodbye.
BOTH Goodbye.

## Interpersonal relations

### Non-verbal communication

It was a rather relaxed interview situation as far as the older brother was concerned. At first he was under the usual degree of constraint, but this disappeared fairly early and the signals the doctor received were friendly. It was not really appropriate for him to accompany the younger child on such an occasion, and this placed him in some difficulty, but he coped with it rather well.

From the child, there was no verbal communication at all until right at the end, when he said 'Yes' to a request that he come again. Favourable relations had been established during the examination procedures described above. It was all done non-verbally; just by his sitting there saying nothing, and the doctor carefully studying his approach. Actions communicated feelings.

Personal space was not a problem to the child, who came and sat down of his own accord right next to the doctor. His brother was close to him on the other side and he was in between, and obviously feeling quite secure.

### Rapport

This developed easily and to a satisfactory level as a result of the doctor's studied attempts to foster it. He spent time and examined the child comprehensively and demonstrated ability to relate to children.

### Confidence

This developed easily built on the rapport. The doctor focused on the prime concern of abdominal pain and displayed knowledge of the range of possibilities, discussing them with the brother and answering his objections. Doctor and brother took part in a short discussion of the possible origins of the pain. Confidence in this situation was of less value than it would have been had a parent been present.

### Agreement

Again, this developed easily on the basis of the generated rapport and confidence.

## General examination

He was not very ill, was alert, intelligent and co-operative, had an expression of interest in the proceedings, and his other general examination findings were normal.

## Summary of clinical evidence

Lower abdominal pain had been recurring over a period of ten months, the latest attack coming on while walking to kindergarten in the morning. He had had some bowel looseness lately, though not on the day when he was seen.

Generally he did not appear at all ill; he walked in hand in hand with his brother, bright, intelligent and alert. He had normal temperature, pulse, respiration and skin characters.

He had a rotational nystagmus present since birth; otherwise regional examination findings were normal.

There was some uncertainty about the quality of parenting, as he had been brought by an older brother.

## Diagnostic processes

### Pattern matching

The pattern of abdominal pain coming on repeatedly over a period of months in a small child following hospitalisation, operation and separation from parents, and precipitated by impending separation, matched closely with the doctor's mental image of abdominal pain in small children subject to anxiety.

### Hypothesis generation and testing

On the basis of the above evidence, the doctor formed the hypothesis that the pain was of psychogenic origin. Testing would only be possible by review over an extended period and observing the outcome.

### Probability

Given the clinical findings, the most probable cause was anxiety.

### Exclusion

*Acute appendicitis*

Recurrent abdominal pain is sometimes a feature

of acute appendicitis, culminating in a severe attack, but the pain on this occasion was not severe and not more severe than previously. In addition, there had been no vomiting. There had been some bowel looseness, which can occur in appendicitis but is uncommon. The child did not appear ill, temperature was 37.0°C, the pulse rate was not raised, and in a relaxed abdomen there was no localised tenderness. Because of these findings, the doctor felt that appendicitis, though not totally excluded, was very unlikely. Review the next day would permit all these findings to be checked to reinforce exclusion of appendicitis.

*Torsion of testis*

Almost certainly his undescended testicle operation would have included fixation to exclude future torsion. Again, the pain in torsion is much more severe and the condition is more common in young adolescents. In addition, there was no abnormality on examination of the abdomen or testes. This condition was really excluded on general examination findings that the patient walked in normally, not in any distress and sat quietly during the interview.

*Urinary tract infection*

This could not be excluded without examination of the urine, which would be done at the next consultation.

### Provisional diagnosis

Psychogenic abdominal pain.

### Provisional social diagnosis

Anxiety in a 3-year-old child brought by a much older brother and with unknown family relationship support.

## Management plan

This was entirely dependent on reassurance of the child, brother and parents, that there was no serious organic disease, and on giving them more insight into the problem. The doctor made definite arrangements to see him again the next day in company with the mother, so that he could discuss the child's condition with her. The doctor also wanted to recheck the child's physical state and to test the urine.

The duration of this consultation was twenty minutes.

## Discussion

In a young child with abdominal pain, it is absolutely essential to achieve a relaxed state of the patient if reliable abdominal findings are to be secured. From the doctor's point of view, the whole of the consultation was shaped by this need.

The doctor set out to get George into a relaxed state by allowing plenty of time for him to become accustomed to the consultation situation, and refraining from making any direct approach in the early stages.

The result was a very good demonstration of the importance of non-verbal communication, as not a word was spoken between doctor and patient throughout the interview until the very end, yet rapport developed extremely well.

Interpersonal relations were of great importance in this interview, not only because of the need for the child to be relaxed, which is always desirable, but also because the family was quite unknown to the doctor. They had not long moved into the area of the practice.

At first the doctor was unaware of the relationship of the two as younger and much older brother. The doctor had thought he was dealing with a young father and his child, and this misconception had its influence on the early stages of the interview.

There were a number of points in the history given by the elder brother which the doctor might reasonably have been expected to follow up, but he did not do so. These included the statement that the child had had some diarrhoea lately, that he kept saying he wanted to go to the toilet and when he got there complained of pain, and that he passed a bit too much in answer to the question about micturition.

The doctor made a conscious decision not to follow these points up because the older brother was obviously somewhat embarrassed by discussion of these physiological details, and the doctor wanted to see the mother with whom he thought he could better go into these matters.

However, this decision of the doctor's not to pursue these lines of enquiry depended on judgment based on history, examination and interpersonal relations that the child was not severely ill.

The doctor judged the probability at this point to be very heavily in favour of a psychogenic etiology. Had the evidence indicated a likelihood of a physical basis, these cues in the history would have been followed up.

The doctor's response to the rotational nystagmus of both brothers is an interesting example of the use of probability in diagnosis in general practice.

The doctor observed that the patient had rotational nystagmus and said, 'He's got wobbly eyes'. The brother immediately responded, 'Yes; same as me', and supplied the medical term, 'It's nystagmus'. This indicated to the doctor that the condition must have been investigated in the older brother, and that he had been reassured about its benign nature, and that the family were not worried about it, either in him or George. So the doctor, too, dismissed the finding as not of significance in this particular instance.

The doctor went to considerable trouble in this examination to secure valid and reliable physical findings and, as stated earlier, this was his major objective at the beginning. He, therefore, deployed all his range of devices for relaxing a young child, and it was successful, but at the expense of time. However, mindful of the serious potentialities of a wrong diagnosis in a child with abdominal pain, he felt the time was well spent, as he ended very confident of the validity of the diagnosis.

★ ★ ★

The full clinical method was applied, though very flexibly, with interview, relationship formation and general examination being carried on, interwoven with regional examination. There was no abbreviation, as the doctor was mindful of the need for great care with children with abdominal pain.

## George—second consultation

*Two days later*

### The record

This revealed that he had not been seen in the intervening two days.

### Interview

DOCTOR Come in. George was with his brother last time.

MOTHER Yes, that's right.

DOCTOR How are things going?

MOTHER Well he still has diarrhoea and is still complaining of pains in the stomach.

DOCTOR How many times has he had diarrhoea today?

MOTHER Once, I think.

DOCTOR Well that's not much diarrhoea is it?

MOTHER No. Well, apparently he was bad at kinder on Thursday (*yesterday*) and when he went home Wednesday afternoon he had it everywhere. It just ran. And apparently Thursday was the same at kinder. He complained of pains in the stomach and the teacher took no notice of him; she had to change singlet, T-shirt, the lot.

DOCTOR Well, what are you doing about diet?

MOTHER I've been trying to keep him off dairy products.

DOCTOR That's right; no eggs, butter, cream, cheese, milk, any of those things. Actually the best treatment is starvation, but you can't starve them for too long.

MOTHER It'd be very hard to starve him. He's eating the whole day.

DOCTOR He's got a good appetite, has he?

MOTHER Oh yes; from the time he gets up till the time he goes to bed, he's eating the whole day.

DOCTOR Well that doesn't sound too bad. Has he had any vomiting?

MOTHER No; just complaining of pains in the stomach.

DOCTOR I wonder if the pain might be due to tension because his brother said . . .?

MOTHER No it hasn't been that long. It's only been this year. I can't see how it could be due to tension because he's almost like an only child, even though he's got two elder brothers. He gets lots of attention; theirs, and mine, and my husband's. You know what I mean?

DOCTOR Sure, yes. But sometimes kids get tension tummy pains even if they're happy, because of excitement. Excitement can cause it too.

MOTHER Yes, yes.

DOCTOR I just thought because it seems to happen on the way to kinder . . .

MOTHER But it could be any time of day. He could walk up to you and say, 'I've got a pain in my stomach'. So the other day when we were going to kinder, I thought I'd come over and make an appointment, because it seemed to be going on for a few weeks.

DOCTOR Did you bring a specimen of his wee?

MOTHER Yes. (*She produced same*)

DOCTOR Well, we couldn't find much wrong with him the other day. We checked him over pretty well . . .

MOTHER I thought it was better to bring him over for a check just in case . . .

DOCTOR Well, you've always got to be careful about appendicitis more than anything else, and he certainly hasn't got that.

MOTHER No? It's not appendicitis, then? My other son had appendicitis, so I know what it's like.

DOCTOR It can be difficult to tell sometimes . . .

MOTHER He was; I didn't believe it at the time.

DOCTOR But this chap doesn't sound like that at all?

MOTHER No, no.

DOCTOR It's something you always have to bear in mind. He's an easy patient to examine, which helps.

MOTHER Yes, he's not bad. Oh, we had a little bit of trouble after he came home from hospital.

DOCTOR Yes, that often happens. Going to hospital and being separated from your parents even only for a day might not seem much to you, but to a child it's important.

MOTHER Yes. And of course it was pretty hectic after he came home, because he was up here all the time . . .

DOCTOR So it was a pretty big experience in his life.

MOTHER Yes.

DOCTOR I'll test his urine . . . Yes, it's normal. And I'll take his temperature. Well, I think he's a pretty healthy little boy really. I think his tummy pain might have a couple of causes. It might partly be due to tension and partly due to a bowel infection giving diarrhoea.

MOTHER Yes, yes.

DOCTOR He hasn't got a temperature now.

MOTHER Well that's good.

GEORGE (*chiming in*) Up or down?

DOCTOR (*to George*) Down.
(*then to mother*) He's very independent for a child not yet 4 years of age. Well, all you can do is wait and see how he gets on. Keep on doing what you are doing already. I can't do any better. The most important thing is to keep him off fat, and you're already doing that.

MOTHER What about bananas?

DOCTOR Oh, he can have those. Bananas are nearly all starch. There's no fat in them. He can have apples too, but I wouldn't give him apricots.

MOTHER Could you just have a look at this rash here? (*She indicated a dry patch of skin on the side of George's face*) It's a bit of eczema and I'm a bit worried about his eyes. If he gets tired it comes out more.

DOCTOR Yes, I'll give you some cream for it.

MOTHER Yes, if you wouldn't mind? You see, I get eczema myself.

DOCTOR Yes, I'll give you some hydrocortisone cream for it; we don't like using the strong creams on the face.

MOTHER Yes, that was what I was a bit worried about.

DOCTOR Has anyone else in the family had diarrhoea?

MOTHER Yes. I've had some myself and some people we visit have had it too. It sounds as though there has been a germ going around.

DOCTOR Yes. Well here's the prescription. I'd put it on three times a day.

MOTHER Thank you.

DOCTOR You were lucky to get into kinder, because there's usually a shortage of places round here.

MOTHER I booked him in as soon as I came to the area twelve months ago, and he got in last December. I thought he needed kinder, with no other kids to play with. He will be going to school next year, and I think they need some kinder first.

DOCTOR Yes, it certainly helps them. Well, let's see him again if he doesn't settle within a reasonable time.

MOTHER Yes; thanks, doctor.

DOCTOR Goodbye.

BOTH Goodbye.

## Interpersonal relations

### Non-verbal communication

At first in this interview the signals were not friendly but neutral. Both mother and doctor wanted to size each other up. Mother was a bit defensive, and the doctor opened up with what could have been seen by her as provocative or accusatory. He said, 'He was with his brother last time'. However, the signals steadily became more friendly from both parties as the consultation proceeded.

Personal space was no problem in this consultation, the mother choosing the chair farthest from the doctor and George sitting between them as in the previous consultation.

### Rapport

None at all in the beginning, but it developed especially after the doctor made it clear that he regarded her as a 'good mother' by saying, 'Keep on doing what you are doing already. I can't do any better'. He also reassured her that it was not appendicitis which really was her main worry.

### Confidence

This grew with rapport, and the mother spontaneously asked for advice on another topic, 'eczema', with which she had had some experience. The doctor displayed knowledge, which she accepted because it tallied with her own experience.

### Agreement

Agreement was readily reached after these exchanges to wait and see with the tummy ache, and to use hydrocortisone cream on the child's face.

## General examination

The doctor decided to go right through the general examination routine because he was dealing with the potentially dangerous condition of abdominal pain in a small child, but in fact the findings were entirely normal.

## Regional examination

The only regional examination done was to palpate the child's abdomen while seated on his mother's knee. This confirmed the absence of guarding, tenderness and rigidity. His urine was also normal.

## Summary of clinical evidence

There had been copious diarrhoea over the previous two days, but no vomiting at any stage. He had still continued to complain of abdominal pain.

He appeared cheerful, contented and alert, was afebrile and looked well.

His abdomen was lax and non-tender, and his urine was normal. There was a dry patch of skin on his face.

His mother presented as caring and competent.

## Diagnostic processes

### Pattern matching

Copious diarrhoea over two days and recent attacks of diarrhoea in family and close acquaintances matched closely with the doctor's mental image of infective diarrhoea.

The fact that mother stated the abdominal pain '. . . could be any time of day. He could walk up to you and say, "I've got a pain in my stomach"' confirmed in the doctor's mind that there was a strong emotional component in the etiology of the pain. This matched with the doctor's experience of children complaining of pain as a means of obtaining a show of affection from parents.

The dry patch of skin on his face conformed to a pattern of minor eczema.

### Hypothesis generation and testing

The above evidence strongly supported the hypothesis of abdominal pain arising from emotional tension, with superimposed infective diarrhoea.

Testing of the emotional factor would only be feasible by review and further observation to check whether progress conformed to the hypothesis.

Bacteriological testing of the infective hypothesis was possible and could be done if the diarrhoea did not soon spontaneously cease.

The eczema hypothesis was to be tested by application of hydrocortisone cream.

### Probability

The doctor judged the probability high that the pain was due to a combination of emotional tension and infective diarrhoea. 'Eczema' also was judged as a probably correct diagnosis.

### Exclusion

Acute appendicitis was excluded by history, general examination and abdominal palpation; urinary tract infection by examine of the urine.

### Diagnosis

Abdominal pain due to emotional tension with superimposed infective diarrhoea and minor eczema of face.

## Management plan

Management included a fat-free diet, more closeness from parents, and hydrocortisone cream for his eczema. The parents were invited to bring him back at any time if they wished for review.

The duration of the consultation was fifteen minutes.

## Discussion

The interview started as a 'straight to the point' exercise by both parties with no 'beating about the bush'. After the doctor had been told that the child 'still had diarrhoea and pains in the stomach', he asked 'How many times today?', seeking to establish the dimensions of the problem. He was also on his guard to refute any suggestion that his failure to prescribe any medicine had been inadequate management at the first consultation. Mother, on her part, was acting aggressively to cover herself against any criticism for not bringing the child herself previously. Thus it started as a joust between them, but non-verbal communication sent by both parties steadily became more friendly as the interview progressed, and they ended by liking each other.

When a child is brought by someone other than the parent, it often raises a question in the doctor's mind as to the quality of parental care. This is especially so when there is no reason given for the absence of the parents. One of the reasons at the back of the doctor's mind in seeking to review this child with a parent present was to assess the quality of care. In this case the doctor was reassured.

Abdominal pain of possible emotional origin necessitates a meeting with one or both parents. It was apparent to the doctor from the non-verbal communication he received from this mother that she had some guilt feelings about not having brought him. However, the doctor gained the impression that she did genuinely believe he was receiving very adequate care.

At this interview, as in the previous one, George just sat quietly listening, and alert. But now there was a non-verbal difference; this time he was obviously happy and contented.

★ ★ ★

Clinical examination was limited to history taking, and regional examination to simple palpation of the abdomen. The main purpose of the interview was to establish a good relationship with the mother.

## Mark—review consultation

### The record

Mark was 6 years of age. He had presented as an acutely ill patient without an appointment and had been seen first, in accordance with standard practice, by the duty sister. She had recorded details that he had been ill for twenty-four hours with a sore throat, and that he had vomited once. Today he had been drowsy, his bowel had opened normally, and micturition was normal, but he had had some abdominal pain earlier.

Accordingly, he had been seen by a doctor, who had found some abdominal tenderness, and the decision had been made that he should be assessed medically later in the day. It was now 8 p.m. and he was accompanied by both parents.

He had a record of viral infections, complicated on several occasions by otitis media, and he had been to an ENT clinic on several occasions.

The family record showed the father to be 31 years and that his family had a history of diabetes mellitus, heart disease and gallstones. It also showed that the father was blind in one eye from trauma.

Mother was 30 years of age and had had two pregnancies. The first child had been large and had presented in posterior position requiring rotation with Kielland's forceps, and the second had been delivered by caesarian section.

The remaining member of the family was a daughter of 12 years who was not present and had been an infrequent attender at the clinic. She had a record of several viral infections, one attack of tonsillitis and one of otitis media.

The family was a stable one, supported by father, who was a good provider, and mother, who was a full-time homemaker.

### Interview

DOCTOR You've been a bit concerned about Mark today?

MOTHER Yes. He hasn't been well and I brought him up to see Dr H. He had a sore tummy. In the last hour or so he said it didn't hurt. He hasn't felt it.

DOCTOR Has he had any vomiting?

MOTHER Once yesterday. Today he's just been lying on the couch and asleep most of the time.

DOCTOR Has he taken Disprin or something similar?

MOTHER Yes; I've just given him paracetamol.

DOCTOR And he's not coughing?

MOTHER He has got a bit of a cough.

DOCTOR More than usual?

MOTHER Oh! Like if he's got a cold.

DOCTOR It's not a big problem?

MOTHER No.

DOCTOR Has he eaten anything today?

MOTHER Yes; he's had a sandwich and Fruit Loops. A little bit of toast. Just whatever he feels like.

DOCTOR Yes; well I better have a look at him. What time did you see Dr H.?

MOTHER Quarter past two.

DOCTOR I'll have a look at the top half of him here on the chair, and then he can take off the rest of his clothes except for his underpants and we'll get him up on the couch. He feels pretty hot, but he hasn't got any spots on him.

FATHER Why has he got goose flesh?

DOCTOR From his fever. That sometimes happens but isn't important. I would say he has 'flu; real 'flu, not just a 'cold'.

Of course, what we have to be careful about is to make sure he's not developing acute appendicitis.

MOTHER That was why I wanted him checked.

FATHER Shouldn't he have some antibiotic?

DOCTOR No. He has only a viral infection, and viruses are not affected by antibiotics. If I gave him antibiotic, there would be a chance of side effects from the drug and no chance of benefit; he might get diarrhoea or vomiting or a rash, and then he would be worse off. It is better to see him again if he is not well.

Sometimes viral infections are followed by bacterial ones, and then, perhaps, he would need some antibiotic. If he gets yellow discharge from his nose, or an earache, or is coughing up yellow from his chest, or you are worried for any reason, I would like to see him again.

FATHER OK. That's fine.

## Interpersonal relations

### Non-verbal communication

Anxiety was evident in both parents more than in the patient, who was fairly relaxed about the whole situation. The mother was most anxious, yet the father was very attentive. Signals were friendly all round.

The family arranged their personal space so that the patient sat on the chair closest to the doctor, the father sat on the chair next to him and the mother stood up, varying her position during the consultation. She began opposite the doctor, separated from him by the desk, and later came to the edge of the couch while her son was being examined. The father remained on his chair throughout.

### Rapport

This developed satisfactorily as the interview went on, and was strengthened by the doctor's full examination and his action in verbalising the fear about appendicitis.

### Confidence

This grew with rapport.

### Agreement

It was agreed to 'wait and see' how the illness progressed on the understanding that the child would be reviewed again next day, or during the night. They were content to accept no immediate action was necessary in the knowledge that he could readily be seen again.

## General examination

The only abnormal finding was a temperature of 38.2°C per axilla and a blocked nose. The doctor decided to do a full examination for comprehensive assessment and to generate confidence in the parents.

## Regional examination

Mark was undressed down to his underpants, but all findings, including urine examination, were normal.

## Summary of clinical evidence

There was a history of abdominal pain earlier in the day, but not in the last two hours. There had been one vomit yesterday, but none today. There had been no diarrhoea and the bowel had functioned normally today. He had not lost his appetite and had eaten snacks during the day. Micturition was normal.

In addition, he had had fever, cough, drowsiness and listlessness today.

Positive examination findings were a temperature of 38.2°C, pulse 90 per minute with a regular rhythm, red pharynx and clear mucus in the nostrils.

Examination of abdomen, including scrotum penis and testes, was normal, and multi-dip testing and micro of urine were normal.

The doctor judged there was a clinically effective level of rapport and confidence by the parents.

## Diagnostic processes

Pattern matching probability and hypothesis all indicated an acute viral infection as the diagnosis; testing was not possible.

### Exclusion

Acute appendicitis was excluded by the history of the cessation of vomiting and pain, normal bowel function and return of appetite, combined with normal abdominal examination findings.

Urinary tract infection was excluded by normal urinary findings.

Torsion of the testis did not fit the pattern presented, but could not be totally excluded as a torsion could have untwisted during the day.

### Provisional diagnosis

Acute viral infection.

### Social diagnosis

The patient was supported by a caring, competent family.

## Management plan

Investigation was not considered necessary beyond routine examination of the urine by chemical tests.

The treatment was conservative, with the parents being advised to take the child home and continue much as they had already been doing. They were advised against giving paracetamol by mouth as there was a small risk of inducing vomiting. They were told about paracetamol suppositories, but advised that in this case they were not necessary. Febrile convulsions were considered very unlikely in a 6-year-old boy who had not previously had one.

The parents were told what to do if they wanted the child seen again. They were invited to ring the clinic and ask to speak to the doctor again if they were worried, but that the condition was not serious and it might not be necessary.

The duration of this consultation was twenty minutes.

### Outcome

He was not seen again for this condition, though records showed that he and the family continued as patients of the clinic.

## Discussion

The first doctor who had seen the child obviously must have been aware of the need to reinforce confidence when he made the decision for the child to be seen later in the day. He had recorded full information in the file, so that the reviewing doctor was able to assess the child's illness in the light of the change in the clinical state in the intervening period.

Early review of children with abdominal pain is the most reliable means of avoiding misdiagnoses, with serious consequences for all concerned. It is especially necessary to be extra careful with acute abdominal pain possibly due to early acute appendicitis. Also, urinary tract infection and torsion of the testis must always be remembered.

Because of the early presentation of these conditions in general practice, doctors must always be ready to make arrangements for review by themselves personally or by a colleague. This review process was put into operation in this case, and it worked well because the first doctor had left adequate documentation of his clinical findings.

The doctor began this interview with the knowledge gleaned from the record that both parents had had some serious health problems themselves in the past, and that this might tend to make them more anxious for their only son's welfare. He wanted to know what their anxieties were, and to this end asked an open question designed to give them an opportunity to voice their concerns. They did not respond rapidly and it was close to the end of the interview before the mother finally voiced her concern about acute appendicitis.

As the doctor knew that parental rapport and confidence were essential in managing the illness, he took special pains to attend closely and to respond appropriately. He also went into some detail in reply to the father's request for antibiotic, as he knew that strong reassurance on this point was necessary. In the event, the advice not to give antibiotic was accepted, probably due to the good level of confidence.

He early had doubts about the possibility of acute appendicitis while taking the history, but resolved to do a complete examination of the child because he wanted to gather comprehensive clinical data and to generate parental confidence. The need for parental confidence was paramount.

★ ★ ★

The full clinical method was deployed because it was a review consultation to exclude acute appendicitis and because of parental anxiety.

An opportunity for education of the parents about the use of antibiotics was seized upon.

## Nancy—first consultation

### The record

Nancy was 9 years old and had a history only of minor viral illnesses.

Family records showed that it was a nuclear family of four persons, including father 49 years, mother 39 years and brother Fred, who was 14 years of age. The father was a regular patient of the clinic for minor illness, including migraine every few months.

The mother had an extensive medical record of chronic illness and operations. She had had two births, both by caesarian section for pre-eclampsia, tubal ligation, hysterectomy and appendicectomy, an accident at work which had resulted in injury to her right arm, and a motor car accident three years previously for which she was still on crutches. It was noted that she had been treated in a Pain Clinic, where her pain had been diagnosed as having a hysterical basis.

Fred had had only minor illness.

The father had a good work record, having been in the same job for more than ten years.

### Interview

*(Nancy hopped in supported on one side by her father and on the other by Fred.)*

DOCTOR *(after inviting them to be seated)* You are Nancy, aren't you? What happened?

NANCY We were at school, the last day of school, and we were doing athletics. I was just going to do a handstand, when one of the other girls did one and fell on me. She had high heels on because it was a casual day, and she went boom on my leg and I couldn't walk.

DOCTOR Right; well, let's have a look at it.

FATHER We thought it would improve, but it hasn't.

DOCTOR Is it getting worse?

NANCY It's getting a bit better every day.

DOCTOR Well that's a good thing. But it's taking a bit longer than expected?

FATHER But you can't walk on it, can you?

DOCTOR Let's have a look at the other one too so we can compare the two together. Can you bend it up? Does that hurt?

NANCY No.

DOCTOR Bend it down. Does that hurt? *(while palpating the dorsum of the sore foot)*

NANCY Ouch! *(This was the first of a series of 'ouchs', which punctuated movements of the mid-tarsal joint and ankle joint. Maximum discomfort seemed to be on palpation of the dorsum.)*

DOCTOR We'd better get it X-rayed.

FATHER I thought it might improve by itself, but you know with Fred . . .

DOCTOR Let's finish with Nancy first. I like to do one thing at a time. I'll see her again after the X-ray.

## Interpersonal relations

### Non-verbal communication

Nancy sent very friendly signals immediately; Fred did too, but somewhat less quickly than his sister. The father was neutral at first, but he slowly became more friendly as the consultation progressed.

Nancy came immediately and sat on the chair right next to the doctor, personal space obviously presenting no problem to her at all. Fred stood up in a somewhat irresolute attitude, and so did the father, who looked rather unrelaxed at first, but he later sat down next to his daughter. He obviously needed to keep some personal space between himself and the doctor.

### Rapport

This was very easily established with Nancy, who obviously wanted to hold the centre of the stage. Fred also wanted to establish friendly relations, but agreed to remain in the background while Nancy had her turn. The father would need to be worked on with some care to build relations.

### Confidence

The doctor set out to get the father's confidence in the expectation that he would be the decision-maker. At first, confidence appeared very tenuous, as the father appeared to have a fixed idea in mind and not to be amenable to other ideas.

### Agreement

Fortunately, both the father and the doctor wanted the foot X-rayed, so there was a measure of agreement from the start. Review arrangements were made without difficulty.

## General examination

She came hopping in on one foot with an air of vitality about her; smiling face and sparkling eyes with otherwise normal findings.

## Regional examination

### Legs

Both legs were examined completely unclothed side by side for comparison and appeared normal; no swelling, bruising or deformity was evident.

There was tenderness over the metatarsal bones of her left foot, and movement of her mid-tarsal joint caused pain. She was also not able to stand on tiptoe with both feet together.

## Summary of clinical evidence

Her left foot had been trodden on two days previously at school and had been too painful to walk on since.

She hopped in looking alert, with smiling face and sparkling eyes, obviously in very good general health.

On inspection and comparison with the other foot, no swelling, bruising or deformity could be detected. She had localised tenderness over the dorsum of her left foot, pain on movement of the mid-tarsal joint and was unable to stand on tiptoe with both feet together.

## Diagnostic processes

### Pattern matching

The clinical findings matched to some degree with the doctor's mental image of cases of fracture of a metatarsal bone. However, due to the absence of swelling, bruising and deformity, the match was not a close one.

### Hypothesis generation and testing

The doctor formed the hypothesis that there was a soft tissue injury only; this would be tested by X-ray.

### Probability

In the doctor's judgment, the evidence pointed to the likelihood of a soft tissue injury only.

### Exclusion

It was essential to exclude fracture of a metatarsal bone.

### Provisional diagnosis

Left foot injury with possible fracture of a metatarsal bone.

## Management plan

It was decided to X-ray the left foot, and this revealed no fracture.

Nancy was to rest, avoid weight-bearing for three days, remain home from school, and then be reviewed.

In discussion with the father, the value of physiotherapy was mentioned as a later option if progress were not satisfactory.

Duration of consultation, including X-ray, was twenty-five minutes.

## Fred—first consultation

### Interview

FRED Yesterday, see, because I was involved in a car accident about five months ago, when I hurt my ribs and had cracked ribs and that . . .

DOCTOR That was five months ago?

FRED Yes. Since then nothing's happened, and then yesterday I was playing and mucking around, and I never felt anything until I got up in the morning; and it was hurting. I couldn't bend or stretch or anything, so I stayed in bed. I stayed in bed all day, and when I got up this morning it was not too bad. It seems like when I strain and do a lot of exercises, next morning it hurts a lot.

DOCTOR Can you take a deep breath? A great big one? What if I press you? (*rib compression produced no discomfort*) It's a little bit tender when I press there? (*pressing the lateral chest wall*)

FRED Yes.

DOCTOR I better have a listen to your chest as well. You haven't had a cold, sore throat, cough, runny nose?

FRED Not lately.

DOCTOR (*addressing the father and indicating the 'sore spot' Fred had complained about*) His lungs are all right; he's just got a sore muscle there.

FATHER (*to Fred*) What was that you were saying about having a sore neck?

DOCTOR Is it sore now? (*with emphasis on 'now'*)

FRED No not now. But it hurts when I muck around.

(*Palpation revealed an area on dorsum of his upper back about the level of T2 near the midline, which he said was painful when pressed upon.*)

DOCTOR (*looking at father*) He's got a sore muscle there too, like the one on the side of his chest.

FATHER Is there any chance of getting him X-rayed?

DOCTOR Yes; I can get him X-rayed, but I don't think it's necessary. But if you want it, I will send him for X-ray. We can't do it here.

FATHER Well I'd like it just in case . . .

DOCTOR But X-ray is not good for you.

FATHER Isn't it?

DOCTOR No. X-rays are not good for you. They can be harmful if you have too many.

FATHER I didn't know that.

DOCTOR Well, if you have too many of them they are not good for you. So it's better not to have X-rays unless you really need them. Quite a lot of people don't like to have X-rays unless there is a very strong reason.

FATHER We're always learning something new.

DOCTOR I don't really think it is necessary for Fred.

FATHER He complains about his side, and he didn't use to complain about anything.

DOCTOR Well, would you like it X-rayed?

FATHER Yes, just to be on the safe side.

DOCTOR All right. Do you want his neck done, or his side, or both?

FATHER Which worries you most, Fred?

FRED The side one is the most . . .

DOCTOR Well, what shall we do?

FATHER I think I'll have both just to be on the safe side.

DOCTOR OK. I would suggest the best thing for him to take is two paracetamol tablets every four hours.

FATHER Actually, I have been giving him aspirin. I think it is better to be on the safe side, because if something develops due to my negligence . . .

DOCTOR Yes. Here is the form, and the easiest way to arrange it is for you to ring up yourself for the appointment tomorrow morning, because there is no one there just now.

## Interpersonal relations

### Non-verbal communication

The doctor received friendly messages from Fred, neutral ones from the father.

Personal space was rearranged during Fred's consultation, as Nancy somewhat reluctantly surrendered her chair next to the doctor and agreed to retire to the background temporarily. The father was on his feet, again not too close to the doctor.

### Rapport

Fred impressed as anxious to develop good relations with the doctor, perhaps even a trifle overanxious. The father was less friendly.

### Confidence

Fred was perfectly ready to accept the doctor's advice, but the father much less so.

### Agreement

The father got his way, which he had been bent on from the beginning. The doctor didn't agree with the decision, but felt it best to accept it. He felt it necessary to comply with the father's wishes if he were to have any influence on the future management.

## General examination

He appeared very well, cheerful and smiling, alert, thickset with some tendency to obesity and with quick active movements; gait was normal, as were other findings.

On the basis of the evidence from the history, general examination and interpersonal relations, the doctor decided to limit regional examination to the chest and spine. Fred was asked to remove his clothes down to his waist and was examined seated, and then standing.

## Summary of clinical evidence

There was a complaint of pain on the right lateral chest wall and in the region of T2 near the midline of his upper back.

He had looked well, cheerful and smiling, with normal gait as he helped his sister into the room when they had first arrived.

Tenderness could not be demonstrated in either site and the location was ill defined in both cases. His movements were free and were not restricted.

His original complaint was rather jumbled and unclear, and he appeared exceptionally anxious to gain attention. Fred's complaints were prompted by his father rather than spontaneous.

## Diagnostic processes

### Pattern matching

The pattern of evidence did not conform to the doctor's mental image of musculo-skeletal injury because of inconsistency of the physical signs.

### Hypothesis generation and testing

The doctor formed the hypothesis that the patient was malingering. Beyond excluding bony injury by X-ray, and clinical review, it would not be possible to test this further.

### Probability

In the doctor's judgment, it was more likely that the symptoms were due to fabrication than injury.

### Exclusion

Bony injury was excluded by X-ray, and other serious pathology by the findings of general and regional examination. Both would tend to be excluded by clinical review.

### Provisional diagnosis

Musculo-skeletal pain.

### Social diagnosis

Both Fred and Nancy were supported by a caring, but apparently overanxious father.

### Management plan

The father was told that aspirin or paracetamol should be used sparingly.

Fred was told that he could do any exercise which was non-painful and that he should try and increase his level of fitness by regular, gradually increasing exercise.

The duration of this consultation was ten minutes.

## Nancy—second consultation

*Eight days later*

#### The record

This showed that Nancy had not been seen at the clinic in the eight days which had elapsed.

Nancy came in with both parents this time and there appeared on general examination to be no change at all in her condition. She was still unable to put her foot to the ground and palpation of the dorsum revealed exactly the same findings as previously.

The doctor decided to get her foot X-rayed again as well as her ankle, which had not been done previously.

In the meantime, her parents were advised to continue the regime of rest.

## Nancy—third consultation

*Five days later*

#### The record

Nancy had not been seen in the intervening five days and her X-rays were reported as normal. Though Fred was not present, the doctor got out his file and discovered that his X-ray result too showed no abnormality.

Nancy hopped in again, supported by both parents.

### Interview

MOTHER What are we going to do with her?

DOCTOR Well, that's what we have to work out, isn't it? Let's have a look. Take your shoes and socks off. Is it getting any better?

MOTHER She says not. She was crying with the pain the other day. I've been noticing her, how she walks, trying not to let her know I'm aware of it. You know what I mean?

DOCTOR Yes.

MOTHER I think it's sore. I can't keep a bandage on her, because every time I touch her she starts screaming.

DOCTOR The X-rays were both all right. (*Examination of the foot proceeded to the accompaniment of a series of 'Ohs!' and 'Ahs!' from the patient, though the doctor was taking extreme care to be gentle.*)
Has she been taking her paracetamol?

MOTHER Yes.

DOCTOR I think I'll send her to the physiotherapist and see what he can do. Then if it doesn't improve, we should put on a plaster to give it complete rest. And if that doesn't succeed, we might need to send her to an orthopaedic specialist. But that should not be necessary if she rests enough. (*The last word spoken with emphasis. The doctor noted that mother was on crutches. 'From a car accident 18 months ago,' she said in response to the doctor's enquiry.*)

MOTHER We kept Nancy home since the accident to make sure of the X-rays, and then it seemed it was hurting her too much to send her to school.

DOCTOR What was expected to be a very simple problem has turned out not to be so simple. I want to see her again next Monday night, and it is very important for her to keep completely off it till then.

## Nancy—fourth consultation

*Two weeks later*

### The record

This showed that the patient had attended for physiotherapy, but had not had any medical consultation in the intervening two weeks.

## Interview

DOCTOR Hello! Well, are we making any progress? Is she visiting the physiotherapist?

FATHER AND NANCY (*in unison*) Yes.

NANCY He put this machine on me and it did a real lot of good for about half an hour, and then it started hurting again and um . . .

FATHER He gave you some exercises too.

NANCY Yes. He told me to do these exercises with my leg, and like he said, I've been doing them. It's still been hurting and today it's been going on and off, on and off, like a machine. And it's been puffed up and gone skinny again, and it was really hurting . . . and . . .

DOCTOR Well, is it any better?

NANCY Just a little.

DOCTOR Well, I'll have a talk to the physiotherapist and we'll perhaps try putting it in plaster if he agrees.

FATHER Actually we have an appointment for tomorrow.

DOCTOR Ah! Well, that will be good, because I will be here too and we can discuss it. We'll see what he thinks. You think it might be a little better?

NANCY Just a little bit. It's been hurting though.

FATHER You were complaining to me this morning that before you put it down on the floor that it's still hurting you.

DOCTOR Well, we'll see what comes out of tomorrow.

FATHER Right, thanks.

BOTH Goodbye.

## Interpersonal relations

Non-verbal communication from both the father and Nancy was now very friendly, and rapport and confidence continued to strengthen. Agreement was readily reached to continue the conservative regime.

## Summary of clinical evidence

At this consultation the findings remained the same except that now Nancy was weight bearing, though with a decided limp.

## Management plan

The patient was to continue with physiotherapy and graduated exercise.

The duration of this consultation was seven minutes.

### Outcome

There was complete resolution after a total of six weeks from injury.

## Discussion

The doctor did discuss the case with the physiotherapist, and agreement was reached to continue the present therapy, which eventually proved successful after six weeks. Most children in this age group would have recovered from such a minor injury in two.

Why did Nancy take so long to get better? There were significant psychological factors which certainly had something to do with it. But also she was a very excitable and effervescent personality, and probably her inability to rest her foot in the early stages was a significant factor in prolonging the disability.

What of the psychological undertones? There was obvious sibling rivalry in the first consultation, which both Nancy and Fred attended, each wanting to hold the stage. It was a case of competing injuries, Nancy's and Fred's, and of whose was the worst and most needed attention from the father.

The father's personality was obviously in part responsible for this disturbed illness behaviour on the part of the children. Repeatedly, he seemed actively to encourage it, reminding them of earlier complaints and appearing to lack insight.

When Nancy said in answer to the doctor, 'It's getting a bit better each day', the father's response was, 'But you can't walk on it, can you?' Earlier, he had said, 'We thought it would improve, but it hasn't'. And in the last consultation, when Nancy said in answer to the doctor's query as to whether it was improving, 'Just a little bit', the father's contribution was, 'You were complaining to me this morning before you put it down on the floor that it's still hurting you'.

Fred was positively encouraged to complain, the father saying, 'What was that you were saying about having a sore neck?' To the doctor it sounded suspiciously as though Fred had forgotten all about it, and had to be reminded.

Earlier, the doctor had the impression that Fred was having some trouble in putting his story together, as it was at first very disjointed. He strongly suspected from this point in the interview that Fred was malingering.

The father had a fixed desire to get X-rays taken, and having achieved this objective, Fred then was allowed to disappear from the scene.

The father's personality impressed the doctor as being rather cold, aloof and rigid. One could not imagine him engaging in a relaxed, loving relationship with his children, and he seemed to have no insight into their manipulation of him. He was obviously anxious for their welfare, overanxious really, and an easy target for the children's manipulative tricks.

The doctor was in the middle of a busy surgery session when this trio walked in, and he wanted to get on with the job and not waste any time, so he was a bit impatient with the father and cut him off in mid-sentence twice. Oddly, this did nothing to impair relationships, the father responding to the doctor's direct approach with increasing rapport over the series of interviews. This came as something of a surprise to the doctor, as did the way the mother presented.

In the record, the mother was depicted as a semi-invalid who had had a series of injuries and illnesses, and ended up at a Pain Clinic with a psychiatric assessment of a hysterical basis for her pain.

In the event, she presented very well as a warm caring, adequate mother. She was also obviously open to manipulation by Nancy, who started screaming whenever the mother tried to touch her foot. However, the emotional detachment of the father was compensated by the emotional warmness of the mother, so that the children ended up not too badly off.

The doctor used some sleight of hand in his examination techniques with both Nancy and Fred, getting both to complain of pain with some inconsistency. He pressed on Fred's lateral chest wall and asked a very leading question as to whether it was sore. Fred promptly responded positively, and later when the doctor re-examined the same area there was no complaint at all. When Nancy's foot was being examined, she was induced to say 'Ouch!' several times in response to no physical stimulus.

In both cases, the doctor judged it better not to point out the exaggeration of symptoms to the parents. At the time, the diagnostic situation was uncertain for Fred, and the doctor judged that Nancy did have some soft tissue injury. To have exposed them might only have impaired relations all round and served no useful purpose.

One aspect worthy of note was that the family always attended after a good deal longer interval of time than arranged by the doctor. The doctor never understood why this happened. It may have been simply difficulty in family logistics.

One further surprise to the doctor was that the parents never took up the suggestion of specialist referral. At first contact, the doctor had expected that the father would want referral early, but in the event neither he nor the mother mentioned it again. The doctor could only speculate as to the reasons.

This series of consultations is an interesting example of family interrelationships and the influence the different personalities had on the response to an injury. Personalities and relationships determined the entire course of events.

★ ★ ★

Clinical method was limited at each contact to general examination and regional examination of the legs for Nancy, and for the only consultation with Fred to general examination and regional examination of his chest and spine. The main concern was to generate adequate relations with all concerned.

## Ron—counselling consultation

Counselling is a feature of many consultations and is to be found in a number of the cases described, but in this one it was the main feature.

### The record

Ron, aged 10 years, had been a patient of the clinic for four years and had attended on seven occasions for minor self-limiting illnesses and several minor accidents, all of which had resolved without difficulty. He had never been in hospital nor suffered from more serious illness. There was a record of allergy to bee sting venom and that he had a booster tetanus toxoid injection two years previously.

His mother had no record at the clinic, though she was in attendance at this consultation, and appeared to be in her mid-thirties.

His father also had no record at the clinic.

### Interview

(*Mother and Ron came in and sat down, with Ron nearest to the doctor.*)

DOCTOR Well, how are you?

MOTHER I want you to check Ron over and tell me what you think about his health. He has been away on a school camping trip and there were some problems with one of the teachers. He was very aggressive towards Ron and attacked him.

DOCTOR What happened?

MOTHER He said Ron had a psychological problem and abused him and poked him in the chest.

I've been on to the principal at the school and said I would sue the school. We had a real shouting match over the phone. So I wanted you to check Ron over to make sure there is nothing wrong with him.

DOCTOR Has he had a 'cold' or any tummy upset?

MOTHER I don't think so, but I would like you to give him a good check-up all the same.

DOCTOR How are you, Ron?

RON OK.

DOCTOR Did you enjoy the camp?

RON Not much.

DOCTOR Why?

RON I didn't like the teacher and some of the other kids.

DOCTOR Can you tell me why?

RON I don't know.

DOCTOR Well, we'd better have a look at you; would you take off everything but your pants and pop up on the couch so I can check you over?

(*Ron complied readily and the doctor examined him from head to toe and found no abnormality.*)

(*to mother*) He seems a normal healthy boy; I can't find anything wrong with him.

MOTHER Thank you. I wanted him checked to make sure he's all right because of the trouble with the school. They said he had a psychological problem. What did they mean by that? I don't think there's anything wrong with him myself, but I wanted you to check him.

(*At this point the doctor decided to continue the interview with the mother only; he suggested that he should talk to her alone, and this was readily accepted by both.*)

DOCTOR You seem extremely anxious and worried, and I wonder why? What does your husband think about it all? Does he get on well with Ron?

MOTHER We are both worried because his sister has 'Parkinson's disease' and he is worried that he might have introduced it into the family. I am worried about all of them.

DOCTOR Are you sure it's 'Parkinson's disease'? Are you sure it's not 'Huntington's disease'?

MOTHER Well, something like that; I'm not sure what it's called.

DOCTOR You need to find out which it is for sure, because there is a lot of difference. Who is looking after your sister-in-law?

MOTHER She is in hospital at present.

DOCTOR I would advise you to contact the hospital and make an appointment to get full information about it. You need to find out for sure.

Also, I think you should make friends with the school, because if you do, it will help Ron. Find out from the hospital first what you can and then make an appointment with the school and tell them about your worries. But you must be friendly to them; if you can't do that, it would be better to keep away.

(*The mother demurred a bit at first at the idea of making friends with the school principal and teacher, with whom she had just had a blazing row, as she was still very angry and not at all inclined to accept such advice.*)

I'm sure you will find them friendly if you adopt a friendly approach to them; it always works in my experience. If you want Ron to get on well at school, you must establish a good relationship with the staff. You need to tell the teachers the reasons for your anxieties, and they are sure to respond well. Ring and make an appointment.

MOTHER All right. But I'll contact the hospital first. (*She appeared more amenable.*)

DOCTOR I would like to see you again next week so we can have another talk about it.

MOTHER All right, I'll do that, thank you. Goodbye.

DOCTOR Goodbye and see you next week.

The duration of this consultation was twenty-five minutes.

**Outcome**

The mother and Ron came next week as arranged. She wanted Ron's throat checked again, and this showed only mild reddening.

She said she had contacted the hospital and it was Huntington's disease; she had made an appointment with a doctor and social worker with the Huntington's Caring Group for counselling.

She also had had a successful interview with the principal and class teacher at the school, which had been very satisfactory; Ron had had a very good week at school.

## Discussion

When this pair walked into the surgery, the doctor immediately picked up the non-verbal message from the mother that she was very angry, anxious and worried, though he had never previously met her. So he encouraged her to ventilate what she was concerned about and co-operated in examining Ron from head to toe, though he did not have any idea as to the source of her worries. He reacted by meeting her immediate expectations of the consultation, hoping that the basic problem would emerge later.

The doctor also picked up the message from Ron's demeanour that he was a bit embarrassed about it all and would have liked not to be involved. As a young pre-adolescent, he remained very peripheral in the consultation. In reality the consultation was with the mother, not Ron.

The basic cause of the mother's anxiety was lack of precise knowledge about Huntington's disease, and her excessive anxiety prevented her from communicating effectively with the school staff.

The mother's anxiety was dealt with by allowing her to ventilate her worries, by checking

Ron over to eliminate the possibility that he had the disease, by setting her on course to get full authoritative information and encouraging her to adopt an effective approach to the school staff.

Listening and discussion diminished anger and anxiety. Prompting the patient to do something, instead of just worrying, also had an effect; action was therapeutic.

★ ★ ★

Clinical method in this consultation was deployed in full so that the mother would be reassured.

# 9 Adolescents

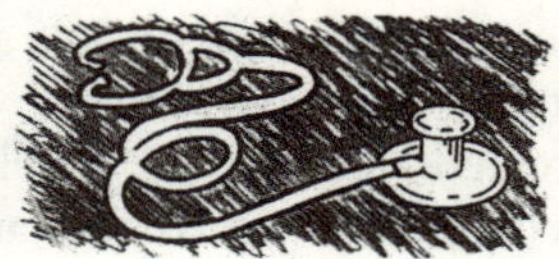

Adolescence extends from 12 to 13 years to the early 20s and is a period of increasing maturity and preparation for independence. Physical growth is very rapid, accompanied by increasing sexual maturity, large nutritional requirements and psychological development; all these processes occur earlier in girls.

Physical health problems include under or over nutrition, fatigue, myopia, scoliosis, kyphosis and acne, and the most serious are accidents and suicide.

## Psychological development

There is a process of increasing appreciation of self as an individual and of relationship with others, of acceptance of physical and sexual identity, of relations with and appreciation of parents, of class identity and the need for decision about a career.

Relations with peers are of great importance and are characterised by sharing of feelings, forming friendships, participation in sports and experiment with relations with the opposite sex as a preliminary to later commitment to an individual.

Though adolescence has been traditionally regarded as a period of turmoil and conflict, recent studies suggest that the majority of adolescents are happy at home and that conflict in adolescence follows conflict in childhood and is followed by conflict in adulthood. Adolescents need the support of their parents, and one of their fears is of premature loss of that support.

Adolescents can behave in a rather adult and mature way when the need arises, as witnessed by the behaviour of the elder brother accompanying George at the first consultation, and the young adolescent accompanying Michael at his first consultation. Both fulfilled the necessary role very adequately.

Rob is an example of an adolescent who has almost achieved maturity and is close to independence, and who is happy at home.

Fred is an example of a young adolescent who is just beginning to test out the possibility of independence, asserting himself as an individual and establishing peer relations in 'mucking around', within a secure, happy, dependent relationship with his family.

## Consultations with adolescents

Generally, success is easily achieved in relating to the adolescent if the approach is the same as to an intelligent adult. The patient will react favourably to being treated as such. Take your history as much as possible from the patient, who is the main storyteller, and only confirm points in doubt with the parent.

The quality of parenting at this age is still very important and good parenting will usually be manifested by encouragement of the patient to speak for him or herself. Inadequate parenting often presents as an inability to appreciate the change in maturity of the adolescent and to modify behaviour accordingly.

Non-verbal communication may succeed in communicating this changed situation to the parent who has not appreciated it previously. Simply speaking to the patient instead of the parent may be sufficient. This, of course, must be well judged and modified according to the parent's reactions.

The parent will in most cases be consumed with anxiety for the welfare of the patient, who may be full of resentment at being treated as a child. Skilfully guided discussion will nearly always resolve this difficulty and allay tensions in both. It is best to have an open and frank three-way exchange; see if you can make both of them laugh.

## Counselling

A prime object of counselling is to establish a good-humoured and tolerant pattern of free communication between parent and adolescent. The ideal is a relaxed atmosphere in the home in which the adolescent has the support of the family while enjoying appropriately increased freedom.

Adolescence is a phase of development with many worries, and at their extreme these are reflected in the suicide rate; hence the great importance of counselling. Worries relate chiefly to relationships with parents, peers, the opposite sex and career prospects.

Counselling of the adolescent should include discussion of the relationship with parents and with the wider community, development of social skills, discussion of sex, future career prospects and any other subject under the sun which the patient wishes to discuss.

Counselling of parents includes advice about their role and the nature of the changes through which their adolescent is passing. Parents may not understand their role fully as models for the adolescent to follow. Parents as teachers transmit values non-verbally to the adolescent as well as factual information, and this may need to be pointed out.

On occasions, it is essential to try and achieve a consultation with the patient alone. The patient may then ventilate worries which cannot be revealed in the presence of the parent. Whether this can happen or not will depend on the doctor having succeeded in generating a sufficient degree of trust, confidence and rapport with the parent, and on parental insight. As always, relationships determine the outcome.

# 10
# Conclusion

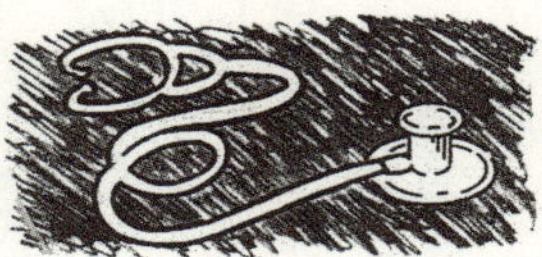

General practice has some inherent difficulties.

Conditions seen range from the most trivial to the most serious.

Serious conditions are randomly distributed among the trivialities.

Trivial conditions are sometimes proffered by the patient as an excuse for visiting the doctor. The real reason may not be revealed unless there is effective rapport.

Trivial conditions may not be trivial to the patient's perception; trivial is a medical value judgment, and there may exist a conflict of perceptions between doctor and patient.

Patients tend to be seen very early in the disease process, and consequently the necessary and sufficient evidence needed for a diagnosis may not be present, and accurate diagnosis impossible at the time of presentation.

Many minor illnesses never cross the diagnostic threshold and spontaneous recovery takes place before they are diagnosable.

Some problems have no solution, but in primary care workers must live with the intractable problem and work out the optimum management; these are problems that no one else has been able to solve.

The number of patients presenting is large and therefore the time available for each is small and must be used to the best advantage.

Good clinical method is required to cope with these inherent difficulties.

Good clinical method is the basis of high quality general practice, and the method set out in this book is a reliable one that allows those new to the field to cope with the unfamiliar situation. Systematic collection of critically evaluated evidence, together with an awareness of the need to develop an effective relationship with the patient, are the main features.

This approach needs to be supported by skill in interview and forming relationships, as well as examination and history-taking skills learned in hospital.

History, general examination and relationships are of overriding importance in good clinical method and are the basis of all consultations, and so have been emphasised in the cases and in the general sections.

An essential feature of general practice is that you are the first and probably the last medically trained person to see the patient. No other doctor is likely to check what you have done, so it is very important for your decisions to be soundly based on systematically collected, critically assessed evidence, according to the scheme outlined. Usually, general practice is first and last contact medicine.

General practice is as intellectually demanding and stimulating as any field of medical work, possibly the most demanding of all because of the range of problems presenting and the fact that pathology presents early.

If you see a patient, apply the clinical method correctly and cure the patient, you can bask in the rosy glow of awareness that you have been very efficient, and the government can bask in the rosy glow of awareness that you have been very cost-effective.

# Appendix 1—Records

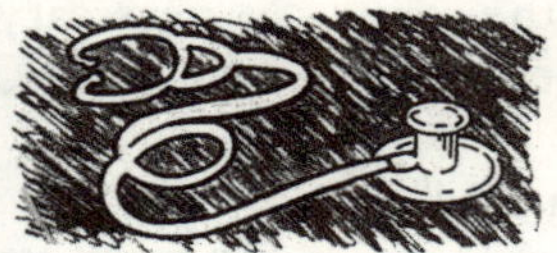

## General practice records

Records in general practice are required for clinical, legal and research purposes, and for preventive health care; the quality of the records tends strongly to reflect the quality of the practice.

## Clinical records

### Acute illness

In acute illness the record documents symptoms, signs, diagnosis, investigations, results of investigations, treatment and the outcome of treatment with specific drugs, including allergy and the outcome of non-drug treatment. There should also be a record of referrals to specialists and hospitals, and the outcome of such referrals. The reasons for the referral should be explicitly stated.

### Chronic illness

In chronic illness there should be similarly a record of symptoms, signs and results of therapy, and this may be continued over a number of years so that the trend of the illness is apparent.

### Once-only history

Present history needs to be taken afresh at each contact, but past history and most of family and social history need to be taken once only, and if time permits, the first contact is the best opportunity.

In present history the dominant symptoms are best recorded in the patient's own words. Words are symbols of a patient's perception of a problem, and if quoted back next time evoke relevant memories and provide the doctor with useful data about progress.

### Be objective

Examination findings should be recorded objectively and as far as possible quantitatively and diagrammatically, and should form a reasonable basis, together with symptoms, for the diagnosis listed in the record.

### Be concise

It is important for progress notes to be concise, with the important symptoms and signs clearly displayed and legible; a mass of verbiage produces only obscurity.

### Preventive health care

For preventive health care purposes, the blood pressure, urine test and weight should be recorded annually, and Papanicolaou smear and intraocular pressures every two years.

### Functional use of record

What does the doctor do when the record is picked up and scrutinised before seeing the patient? Experienced doctors look first at the name and whether the patient is known to them, the date of the last attendance and the nature of the problem at that time. Note will also be taken of the treatment given and the outcome when recorded, who is the regular doctor, and the patient's age. Check date of birth to ensure the file is the correct one; two people of the same name may be patients of the practice, perhaps at the same address.

Then the front-page summary is scanned for the main past problems, and the reports summary page to check the most recent entries.

During the consultation there is normally further checking of the exact nature of previous presenting problems to see if they are similar to the current one, further close checking of reports before deciding whether to order further tests, and a check is always made of allergies in the front-page summary before ordering any medication.

## RACGP record system

This record system used in the author's practice consists of an A4 manilla folder and three types of record sheet—a front-page sheet of medically important facts about the patient called the Health Summary, Progress Notes, which are a day-to-day record of patient attendances, and a Reports Summary sheet.

The folder is designed to contain one patient's record with a unique number, and is filed in accordance with the number. The folder also has provision for linkage with files of other members of the family and for serial recording of blood pressure, urine testing and weight. These last features are designed to promote preventive health care.

## Problem orientation

The RACGP record is designed to permit problem orientation of records, both in the Health Summary sheet and Progress Notes.

This is of most value in chronic illness, less in acute illness, unless there are recurrent bouts of the same acute illness.

The design of the Progress Notes encourages recording of objective evidence for each problem; each problem is recorded with its own set of symptoms, signs, diagnosis and plans for management, and is given a number which is also recorded on the front page of the Health Summary sheet. The management of each problem is also recorded very briefly on the Health Summary sheet and brought up to date as necessary.

The RACGP record is illustrated in Figures A1.1, A1.2 and A1.3.

## Correspondence file

Correspondence about patients is best kept in a separate system of filing cabinets. In addition, if the treating doctor wishes, reports from specialists, hospitals and investigations can also be kept. But most reports are most usefully summarised in chronological order in the Reports Summary sheet in the patient's history.

## Communication really is vital

Communication of clinical details about patients between doctors in the same practice, between doctors and paramedical workers, and between doctors and specialists and hospitals is vital to the patient's best interests. Legibility in this context assumes special importance; it is hard to exaggerate its importance, and the ultimate in legibility is for the record to be typed.

## Photocopying

If the Health Summary and Reports Summary sheets are typed, a photocopy of these and a note about the current illness and the reasons for referral provide excellent communication at minimum cost.

## Medico-legal requirements

Requests from solicitors for reports on patients are very frequent, and for this purpose it is essential to keep full clinical records, in addition to copies of all letters sent, as well as the originals received, together with consent forms signed by the patient authorising release of information.

## Certificates

Certificates written for a patient should be documented in the history so that the doctor has a record of what has been written.

RACGP HEALTH RECORD

**Health Summary**

| Date Commenced | CATEGORY & NUMBERS | SURNAME | RECORD NUMBER |
|---|---|---|---|
| | M.C. 0000 00000 0 | JAMES | 57248 |
| | | GIVEN NAMES: Rita | |

| | | | |
|---|---|---|---|
| DATE of BIRTH: 3.5.76 | COUNTRY of BIRTH: Australia | ADDRESS: 7 Wilson Street, East Melbourne | |
| MARITAL STATUS: S | SEX: F | NEXT of KIN: Father - Ken | |
| OCCUPATION: Student | | RELIGION | |
| EMPLOYER or SCHOOL: High School | | BLOOD GROUP / Rh | PHONES: Home 987 6543 Bus. |

**SOCIAL AND FAMILY HISTORY**

Mother D.O.B. 17.8.51 - asthma
Father D.O.B. 3.10.49 - well
Sister (Julie) D.O.B. 2.4.78 - asthma
Brother (Ian) D.O.B. 1.9 80 - well

**PROBLEM LIST**

| Date | No. | Past Problems | Code |
|---|---|---|---|
| 1984 | | Recurrent cystitis | |
| 1984 | | Reimplantation ureter for reflux (RCH) | |

**IMMUNISATIONS**

| Year | Type |
|---|---|
| 1976 | Triple antigen |
| 1976 | Sabin |
| 1977 | Measles Mumps Triple antigen |
| 1981 | C.D.T. Sabin |
| 1988 | Rubella |

**ALLERGIES & SENSITIVITIES**

| Year | Antigen | Type and Severity |
|---|---|---|
| | Nil known | |

| Date | No. | Active Problems (from commencement date) | Code | MANAGEMENT | Date Resolved |
|---|---|---|---|---|---|
| 1985 | 1 | Urinary tract infection | | Nitrofurantoin 50 mg b.d | 1985 |
| 1985 | 2 | Irritable right hip | | Rest and paracetamol | |

RACGP (C) 02/85

**Fig. A1.1** *RACGP Health Summary sheet. Reproduced with permission of The Royal Australian College of General Practitioners.*

PAGE No. 1

# Progress Notes

SURNAME JAMES | RECORD NUMBER 57248
GIVEN NAMES RITA

| DATE | Prob No. | SOA | FINDINGS: Subjective, Objective, Assessment | DTI | PLANS: Diagnostic, Therapeutic (including medication), Information |
|---|---|---|---|---|---|
| 3.3.85 | 1 | S | mother wants Rita to have urine test - | | mother reassured - |
| | | | last year had a reimplantation of | | for a further M.S.U.* |
| | | | ureters for reflux and has recently | | in one week |
| | | | been on nitrofurantoin - feels well - | | |
| | | O | urine test showed albumen + | | |
| | | | nitrite - ve | | |
| | | A | no U.T.I. now | | |
| 20.3.85 | 1 | S | occasional scalding | | M.S.U. sent to |
| | | O | N.A.D. | | laboratory |
| | | A | dysuria N.Y.D. | | |
| 27.3.85 | 1 | S | well - came for results | | M.S.U. N.A.D. |
| | | S | sore eyes for one day | | advice re eyes |
| | | O | eyes N.A.D. | | |
| 5.6.85 | 2 | S | fell downstairs one week ago - R leg | | rest |
| | | | now sore - limping - not in any | | paracetamol |
| | | | distress - | | X-ray pelvis + |
| | | O | ext. rotation of R leg ?may limited - | | R femur |
| | | | left leg OK. | | |
| | | A | painful R. hip N.Y.D. | | review tomorrow |
| | 1 | S | for another M.S.U. | | M.S.U. sent |
| 6.6.85 | 2 | S | R leg still sore | | |
| | | O | same | | ? diagnosis |
| | | A | painful R hip | | review at hospital |
| | 1 | A | U.T.I. | | nitrofurantoin 50 mg |
| | | | | | b.d. |
| | | | | | see specialist again |
| 1.7.85 | 1 | | phone from specialist | | leave off medication |
| | | | | | for 4 weeks then |
| | | | | | M.S.U. |
| 10.2.86 | 1 | S | well - for rpt M.S.U. - mother to | | M.S.U. sent |
| | | | phone for result - | | |
| 29.4.86 | 1 | S | wants M.S.U. | | M.S.U. sent |
| 28.5.86 | | S | sore foot 3 weeks | | cryotherapy |
| | | O | papillomata on sole | | |
| | | A | plantar warts | | |
| 14.6.86 | | S | foot still sore | | rpt cryotherapy |



**Fig. A1.2** *RACGP Progress Notes sheet. Reproduced with permission of The Royal Australian College of General Practitioners.*

PAGE No.

# Reports-Summary

RACGP HEALTH RECORD

SURNAME | RECORD NUMBER

GIVEN NAMES

| DATE | |
|---|---|
| 23.3.85 | PATHOLOGY: No 12345 M.S.U.* N.A.D.+ |
| 6.6.85 | RADIOLOGY: No 34078. Pelvis and right femur: N.A.D. |
| 6.6.85 | PATHOLOGY: No.668050. (6G24). - Urine - M.S.U. E.coli 100 000 orgs/ml. Sulphafurazole RESISTANT, Co-trimoxazole RESISTANT. |
| 10.6.85 | CHILDRENS HOSPITAL: General Clinic/Emergency - Pain right knee - resolved. Limp - resolved. Some limitation abduction right hip - improving. Irritable hip. U.T.I. - E. coli. |
| 25.6.85 | PATHOLOGY: No. 668163 (GN16) - M.S.U. Protein + Leucocytes 70. Erythrocytes 30. Scanty insignificant growth 5000 orgs/ml. PROTEINURIA AND HAEMATURIA. |
| 26.7.85 | MR ROBERT: I reimplanted her left ureter by an anti-reflux technique on 13.8.84 and her early post-operative progress was uneventful. She did however have a recurrence of U.T.I. about Christmas time, but nothing since and has remained off maintenance chemotherapy. The recent Nuclear Scan at the R.M.H. (copy of report enclosed) is mildly disappointing in some respects, but reassuring overall. There is excellent renal function, with no hint of post-operative ureteric hold-up or stenosis, and only one fleeting episode of reflux was seen on either side, and only during micturition. Previously, she refluxed freely during passive filling of the bladder as well as during voiding. With these findings there is no clear-cut indication to put her back on maintenance chemoprophylaxis, but you need have little hesitation in doing so if she has further recurrence of U.T.I. which, in your view, are too frequent or severe. If this should happen, I would welcome an opportunity to see her again, at your request, with a view to cystoscopy. |
| 15.8.85 | PATHOLOGY: No. 722451. M.S.U. N.A.D. |
| 10.2.86 | PATHOLOGY: No. 822409. M.S.U. N.A.D. |
| 29.4.86 | PATHOLOGY: No. 876319. M.S.U. N.A.D. |
| 9.7.86 | PATHOLOGY: No. 943050. M.S.U. N.A.D. |
| 6.8.86 | PATHOLOGY: No. 994147. M.S.U. N.A.D. |

* Mid-stream specimen of urine
+ No abnormality detected





Reports-Summary

**Fig. A1.3** *RACGP Reports–Summary sheet. Reproduced with permission of The Royal Australian College of General Practitioners.*

## Freedom of information

The freedom of information legislation does not apply to the records of private practice but does to records in a health centre, and patients of the centre are entitled to obtain copies of the record if they wish. In the case of a patient with a psychiatric illness, there is a provision that, if material in the file is considered likely to adversely affect the patient, a medical practitioner nominated by the patient must be allowed access to the file and inform the patient appropriately of the contents.

## Research

Data recorded in general practice files is a very valuable basis for research into many aspects of common illness.

ICHPPC-2-Defined (International Classification of Health Problems in Primary Care) is a system of coding for presenting problems in general practice, with criteria for coding for most problems. It provides a potential for research to determine the best treatment for common illness. (See Appendix 2—Problems.)

# Appendix 2—Problems

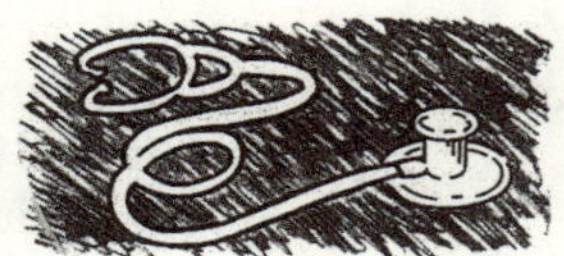

This section documents the very large range of illness and related problems that present to general practitioners.

## Presenting problems

The problems that may present to a doctor in general practice number over 370 according to ICHPPC-2-Defined (International Classification of Health Problems in Primary Care-2-Defined). 'Defined' means that criteria for most problems are included.

The problems in the classification include diagnoses, presenting symptoms and signs that have not yet been diagnosed, and a very wide range of social problems and administrative procedures that call for the doctor's participation.

In the third edition, many of the problems have established criteria for coding, which is aimed at producing uniformity of coding between different observers.

The ICHPPC-2-Defined classification is intended principally as a research tool, permitting comparative studies between different practices worldwide.

Problems or 'illnesses' are classified into eighteen major groups, which are set out below:

1. Infective and parasitic diseases.
2. Neoplasms.
3. Endocrine, nutritional and metabolic diseases.
4. Diseases of blood and blood-forming organs.
5. Mental disorders.
6. Diseases of the nervous system and sense organs.
7. Diseases of the circulatory system.
8. Diseases of the respiratory system.
9. Diseases of the digestive system.
10. Diseases of the genito-urinary system.
11. Pregnancy, childbirth and puerperium.
12. Diseases of the skin and subcutaneous tissues.
13. Diseases of the muscolo-skeletal system and connective tissue.
14. Congenital anomalies.
15. Perinatal conditions.
16. Physical signs, symptoms and ill-defined conditions not otherwise specified or not yet diagnosed.
17. Accidents, poisonings and violence.
18. Supplementary classifications.

**Example**

The first child case presented in this book, that of 'Con', is coded as follows according to ICHPPC-2-Defined:

138 466 Bronchitis, bronchiolitis, acute incl. bronchitis NOS (not otherwise specified); tracheobronchitis.

The criteria listed for inclusion of a condition in this rubric require both of the following features to be present:

(a) cough;
(b) scattered or generalised abnormal chest signs—wheeze, coarse or moist sounds.

ICHPPC-2-Defined also includes a note that bronchiolitis in infants may be present as dyspnoea and obstructive emphysema without wheeze, moist sounds, fever or sputum, and alternative classifications are quoted for consideration.

These include:

133 460 Upper respiratory tract infection
144 493 Asthma
269 7860 Wheezing
270 6862 Cough.

ICHPPC-2-Defined mentions an important point that the coding is for conditions as they present early in the pathological process, and that conditions seen later would certainly be coded somewhat differently in some cases. It is a coding of presenting problems.

## Survey

The results of a survey of problems by five doctors in the author's practice are summarised in Figure A2.1.

Patients in the survey were seen at Deer Park Community Health Centre.

They were consecutive patients of five participating doctors, but were not a total of the patients attending the practice in that time. Participating doctors each coded consecutive patients for a week, but not concurrently.

This ratio of male to female patients is usual in surveys in general practice. It is also usual for many patients to present with more than one problem.

The population served is a very young one, with many young married families with young children.

* * *

It is because of the very wide range of problems presenting in primary care, allied to the early presentation of pathology, that clinical method assumes such great importance to the general practitioner.

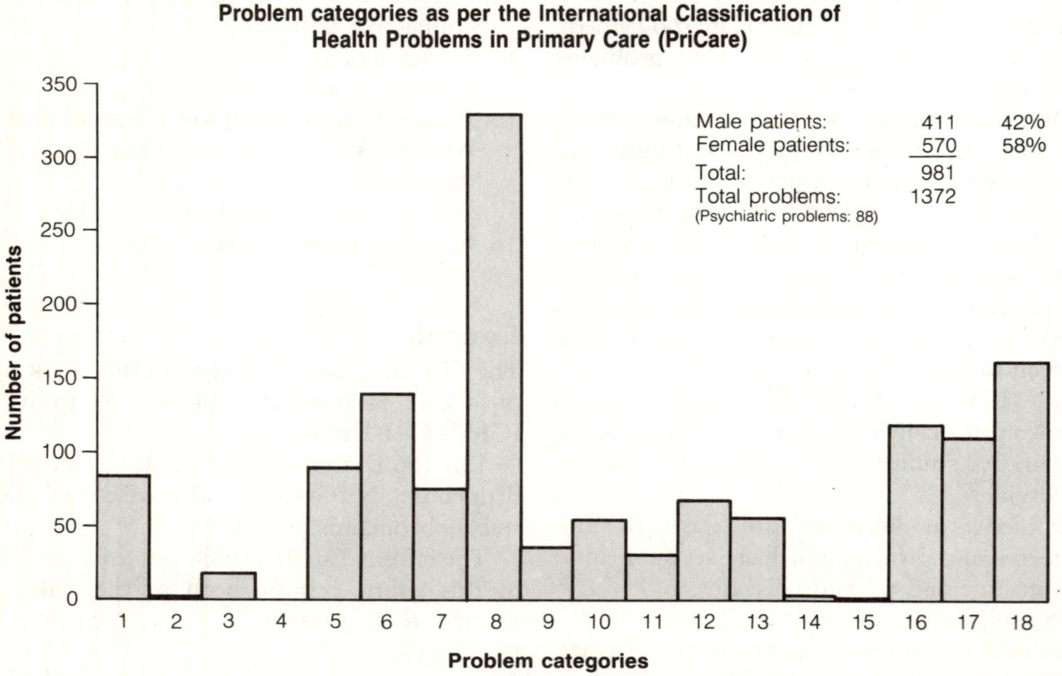

**Fig. A2.1** *Deer Park Community Health Services patients seen between 8.10.79 and 21.1.80.*

# Appendix 3—Clinical checklist

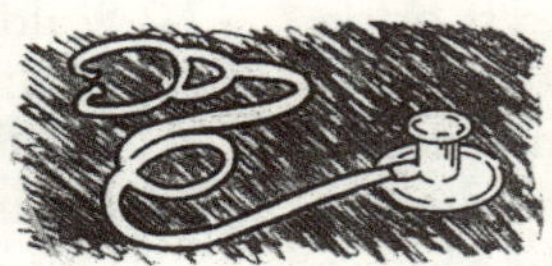

## Relationship with patient

*Non-verbal communication (NVC) commences between you and the patient from the moment the patient walks into the surgery. Facial expression, tone of voice, appearance and dress, bodily movement and gestures all send messages to the doctor. Are the messages friendly, neutral or unfriendly?*

*Personal space is most important at the commencement of the interview; where does the patient sit in relation to you?*

### 1. Present history

1.1 Name.
1.2 Age.
1.3 Address.
1.4 Marital state.
1.5 Occupation.

*How serious is the patient's concern judged from the NVC?*

*What does the NVC tell you about the patient's emotional state?*

### 2. Presenting complaint

2.1 Complaint and duration.
2.2 Previous similar attacks.

*Is the NVC from the patient consistent with the complaint?*

*What are you, the doctor, feeling towards this patient and what kind of NVC are you sending to the patient? Rapport development largely occurs early in a consultation; this is the time to work on it.*

*Are you making appropriate eye contact, attending closely and appearing to do so, and making appropriate responses, both verbal and non-verbal?*

*Has the patient made an attempt to generate rapport with you? Smiled at you and greeted you as a friend, perhaps, if known to you, or asked how you are or, if you've been away, whether you had a good holiday?*

*Or is the patient entirely wrapped up in personal concerns and making little or no attempt to relate to you as an individual?*

*At times patients adopt too personal an approach, which is the direct opposite of the self-centred patient. You may feel the need to distance yourself from this type of patient approach.*

*Very occasionally a patient may seek to sit closer to you than is comfortable, and you may feel obliged to move away a little, or as an alternative get up and walk up and down for a moment or two. The doctor feels the need for personal space as does the patient.*

### 3. Most relevant system

*Systematic enquiry commences with the one most relevant to the presenting symptoms; continue according to the following schedule but not necessarily in the same order.*

*While the patient is telling his or her concerns, you must attend very closely and appear to do so, making apt responses.*

### 4. Respiratory system and ENT

4.1 Nose; whether obstructed or not and the character of any discharge; clear mucus, purulent or bloodstained.

4.2 Throat; whether sore on swallowing and the location of soreness.
4.3 Ears; any deafness, buzzing, pain or discharge.
4.4 Headache; its location, character and whether modified by posture or movement.
4.5 Shortness of breath; whether at rest or on exertion and if accompanied by wheeze.
4.6 Cough; frequency, time of occurrence, if associated with pain, whether productive of sputum or not, and whether the sputum is clear, purulent or bloodstained.
4.7 Enquire about smoking in adults.
4.8 Pain in the chest; type of pain, when and where, and what physiological functions modify or precipitate it.

**5. Cardiovascular system**

5.1 Shortness of breath; at rest, during or after exertion, at what time?
5.2 Pain in the chest; type, when, where and what physiological functions modify or precipitate it?
5.3 Swelling of ankles, legs, thighs, lower abdomen and sacral region, and whether it fluctuates at different times of day.
5.4 Palpitations; what factors, if any, precipitate them?
5.5 Smoking; how much?

**6. Alimentary system**

6.1 Appetite.
6.2 Dysphagia.
6.3 Indigestion; this varies from heartburn to severe pain.
6.4 Anorexia, nausea, vomiting; character of vomitus.
6.5 Diet; does it include the basic essentials and is there any specific intolerance for any food?
6.6 Tobacco, alcohol and drug use.
6.7 Weight, including any change.
6.8 Bowel function; constipation, diarrhoea should be enquired about and also character of stools and whether any blood.
6.9 Abdominal pain; temporal and spatial distribution and physiological correlations.

*Obtaining useful information on smoking, alcohol and drug use depends heavily on rapport. What does NVC convey?*

**7. Renal system**

7.1 Frequency of micturition.
7.2 Scalding.
7.3 Pain; temporal and spatial distribution and physiological correlation.
7.4 Haematuria.
7.5 Dysuria; stream characteristics, nocturia, polyuria, stress incontinence.

**8. Reproductive system**

8.1 Menses; normal or disturbed functional pattern.
8.2 Vaginal discharge and characteristics.
8.3 Sexual function.
8.4 Urethral discharge.

**9. Central nervous system**

9.1 Sleep; quantity and quality, and any disturbance from the normal pattern.
9.2 Headache; temporal and spatial distribution and physiological correlations.
9.3 Eye symptoms.
9.4 Faints, fits or falls.
9.5 Giddy turns, including description from a close observer if possible.
9.6 Numbness and tingling sensations.
9.7 Weakness.
9.8 Buzzing in ears.
9.9 Visual disturbances and characteristics.
9.10 Paralysis.

*Subjective CNS symptoms are extremely common; NVC is particularly important in assessing them.*

**10. Musculo-skeletal system**

10.1 Pain; temporal and spatial distribution and physiological correlations.
10.2 Weakness; loss of function.
10.3 Swellings.
10.4 Deformities.

**11. Endocrine system**

11.1 Tiredness, weakness.
11.2 Nervousness.

11.3 Weight change.
11.4 Thirst.
11.5 Polyuria.

**12. Haemopoietic system**

12.1 Tiredness.
12.2 Weakness.
12.3 Shortness of breath.
12.4 Bleeding or bruising.

*Vague symptoms are extremely common and NVC provides valuable additional data.*

**13. Past history**

13.1 Other illnesses.
13.2 Accidents, operations, hospitalisations.
13.3 Obstetric history.
13.4 Allergies; especially to drugs.
13.5 Immunisations.
13.6 Present drug medication.
13.7 Previous similar illness—reiteration.

**14. Family history**

14.1 Parents' health including hypertension, diabetes mellitus, asthma, 'nerves', arthritis, epilepsy.
14.2 Brothers and sisters and their state of health.
14.3 Children and their state of health.

*Comprehensive enquiry about past and family history can strongly build rapport and confidence.*

**15. Social history**

15.1 Health of spouse.
15.2 Home life; is it relaxed and happy?
15.3 Marriage; quality of relationship.
15.4 Children; their relationships with sibs and parents.
15.5 Extended family relations.
15.6 Work; relations, hours, is it too heavy or are the conditions harmful? Is there contact with noxious materials?
15.7 School; relations with peers and teacher?
15.8 Creche or kindergarten; is it satisfactory?
15.9 Housing; quality and cost.
15.10 Leisure; are there adequate social contacts? Does the patient get sufficient exercise?

*Is the patient happy to talk about home and family and social life or restrained? NVC will tell you.*

**16. General examination**

16.1 Illness.
16.2 Intelligence.
16.3 Co-operation.
16.4 Expression.
16.5 Build and weight.
16.6 Posture and movement.
16.7 Temperature.
16.8 Pulse.
16.9 Respiration.
16.91 Blood pressure.
16.92 Skin; pallor, jaundice, cyanosis, pigmentation, presence or absence of rash, hair.
16.93 Swellings.
16.94 Deformities.

*Much of the early general examination will have been communicated by NVC.*

## Clinical decision

*On the basis of data from history, general examination and relationship, how much psychological and regional examination is required and acceptable to the patient.*

**17. Psychological state**

17.1 General appearance and behaviour.
17.2 Thought processes—talk.
17.3 Mood.
17.4 Delusions.
17.5 Hallucinations.
17.6 Obsessions.
17.7 Orientation.
17.8 Memory.
17.9 Attention and concentration.
17.91 General information.
17.92 Intelligence.
17.93 Insight and judgment.
17.94 Personality; are there any traits evident that suggest obsessional, schizoid, hysterical or paranoid behaviour?
17.95 Sociopathy? Is the patient unduly passive or aggressive?

*Much of this will already have been communicated by NVC.*

*Regional examination requires the patient to surrender completely his or her personal space; is the NVC signalling compliance?*

## Regional examination checklist

### 18. Head

18.1 Scalp and hair.

18.2 Skull shape and fontanelles in infants.

18.3 Face; general inspection including 7th nerve function, exophthalmos, endophthalmos.

18.4 Eyes; periorbital tissues, lids, lashes, pupils and reactions, corneae, conjunctivae, retinal inspection, acuity of vision, intraorbital pressures (Schiotz tonometer), and movements in H pattern.

18.5 Ears; inspection of external ear, palpation of pre- and post-auricular areas for tenderness, presence or absence of pain on traction of external ear, inspection of drums by auriscope, characteristics of any discharge.

18.6 Nose; whether obstructed or not, whether any discharge and its characteristics if present, inspection of anterior nares.

18.7 Mouth; lips, gums, teeth, tongue and its movement, breath, palate, mucous membrane, fauces and tonsils, and whether any post-nasal discharge present or not and its characteristics.

18.8 Cranial nerves; motor function by observing the movements of face, eyes, lips, tongue, pharynx, sternomastoids and trapezii. Sensation of face tested with pinprick or cotton wool. Taste and smell are rarely tested in general practice. Deafness and visual defect are tested in the surgery to a limited extent. Vestibular function tested by head movements.

### 19. Neck

19.1 Inspection; note presence or absence of swelling of thyroid, lymph glands, parotids and submandibular salivary glands, and condition of skin. Note thyroid outline during swallowing.

19.2 Palpation; note whether lymph glands enlarged or tender, thyroid enlarged smoothly or nodular or not enlarged.

Trachea; midline or not.

Movements of neck; flexion, extension, lateral flexion and rotation, range of movement and whether pain free, and power.

19.3 Auscultation; arteries and thyroid for murmurs.

### 20. Chest—anterior aspect

20.1 Inspection.
Type of chest.
Symmetry.
Rate, depth and character of respiration.
Pulsations.
Distended vessels.
Respiratory movements—equality.
Breasts.
Skin.

20.2 Palpation
Breasts.
Apex beat.
Trachea.
Pulsations.
Respiratory movements—equality.
Voice sounds (vocal fremitus).
Trunk movements; range and whether pain-free.
Chest wall; presence or absence of tenderness.
Skin; sensation.

20.3 Percussion.
Lungs, heart, liver.

20.4 Auscultation.
Breath sounds.
Adventitial sounds.
Voice sounds (vocal resonance).
Heart sounds and murmurs.
Friction rubs; pleural, pericardial.

### Chest—posterior aspect

20.5 Inspection.
Spine; deformities. Type of chest configuration.
Symmetry.
Movements; equality.
Skin.

20.6 Palpation.
Spine; movements, tenderness.
Voice sounds (vocal fremitus).
Skin sensation.

20.7 Percussion.
Lungs.

Spine; with closed fist over spinous processes for deep tenderness.

20.8 Auscultation.
Breath sounds.
Adventitial sounds.
Voice sounds (vocal resonance).

**21. Abdomen**

21.1 Inspection.
Size, shape, symmetry.
Movements; respiration, pulsations, peristalsis, impulse with cough at hernial orifices. Marks; dilated vessels, scars, umbilical contour, hair distribution, stretch marks, skin rash.
Penis, scrotum.

21.1 Palpation.
Guarding, tenderness, rigidity.
Splashes, fluid thrill.
Viscera.
Masses.
Inguinal lymph glands.
Hernial orifices; impulse on coughing while standing.
Skin; sensation, superficial abdominal reflexes. Scrotum, testes, epididymes.
Vaginal examination; digital and speculum.
Rectal examination; digital and speculum.

21.3 Percussion.
Hyper resonance. Dullness; liver, spleen, bladder, masses.

21.4 Auscultation.
Bowel sounds, foetal heart.

**22. Arms**

22.1 Inspection
Both together in same posture; muscular contours, symmetry, skin, nails and hair.
Active movements.

22.2 Palpation.
Tenderness.
Pulse, arteries, blood pressure.
Lymph glands.
Joints; pain-free range of movement.
Power, tone, movements and co-ordination, reflexes and sensation.

**23. Legs**

23.1 Inspection.
Both together in the same posture; muscular contours, skin, nails, veins, oedema.
Active movements; walking, sitting, standing.

23.2 Palpation.
Tenderness.
Pulses; femoral, popliteal, dorsalis pedis, posterior tibial arteries.
Lymph glands.
Joints; pain-free range of movement.
Power, tone, movements and co-ordination, reflexes and sensation.

**24. Pathology laboratory**

24.1 Sputum; macro and culture.
24.2 Vomitus; macro.
24.3 Stools; macro, culture, micro.
24.4 Urine; macro, micro, chemical test, culture.

**25. Personal diagnosis**

*Ask yourself the following questions before the end of the consultation:*

1. *Why did this patient come today?*
2. *What are the patient's expectations of this consultation?*
3. *How will this illness affect the patient, his or her family, work and leisure?*
4. *Is this patient likely to comply with therapy?*

# Appendix 4—Clinical perspectives

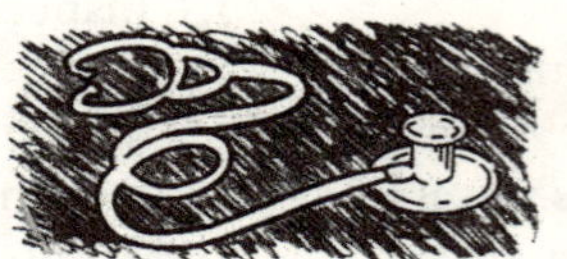

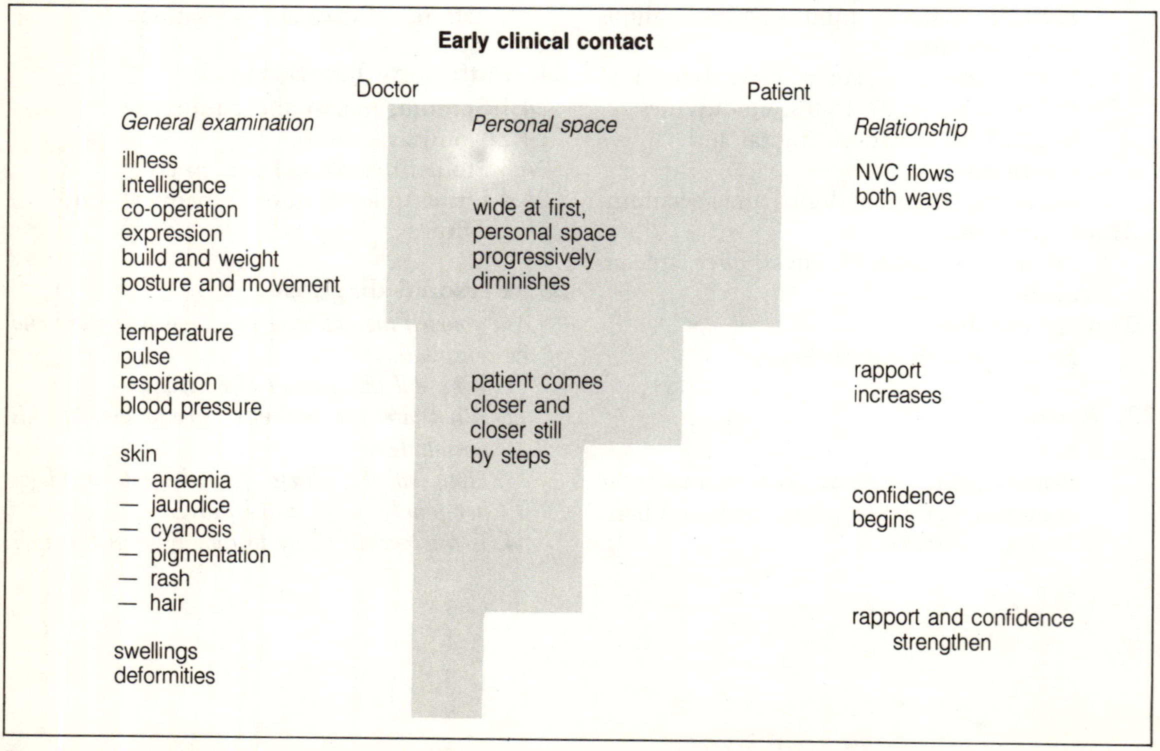

**Early clinical contact**

Doctor — Patient

| *General examination* | *Personal space* | *Relationship* |
|---|---|---|
| illness<br>intelligence<br>co-operation<br>expression<br>build and weight<br>posture and movement | wide at first,<br>personal space<br>progressively<br>diminishes | NVC flows<br>both ways |
| temperature<br>pulse<br>respiration<br>blood pressure | patient comes<br>closer and<br>closer still<br>by steps | rapport<br>increases |
| skin<br>— anaemia<br>— jaundice<br>— cyanosis<br>— pigmentation<br>— rash<br>— hair | | confidence<br>begins |
| swellings<br>deformities | | rapport and confidence<br>strengthen |

**Fig. A4.1** *This is the most common pattern. Sometimes the doctor moves more than the patient.*

**Critical evaluation**

*The record*

What is the quality of the evidence for any diagnosis quoted in the record?

*Patient's story*

Is there any contradiction:
— in what is spoken?
— with the record?
— with the patient's NVC?

*Examination*

Are signs consistent or variable?

*In summary*

Never believe what the patient tells you and never disbelieve it—
look for other evidence to confirm or refute it.

**Fig. A4.2**

**Interview techniques**

*Verbal communication*

| | | |
|---|---|---|
| 'open' questions | → | undirected, wide-ranging response |
| 'closed questions' | → | directed monosyllables |
| responding | → | shows interest and concentration |
| repetition | → | amplifies undirected information |
| comment on NVC | → | stimulates more undirected information |

*Non-verbal communication*

| | | |
|---|---|---|
| attending | → | shows you are listening |
| eye contact | → | shows you are interested |
| bodily attitude | → | leans forward, shows you are concentrating |
| expression | → | shows emotional response |
| mood | → | empathy with patient |
| tone of voice | | |
| interrogatory | → | more undirected information |
| exclamatory | → | |

**Fig. A4.3**

**Clinically effective relationship**

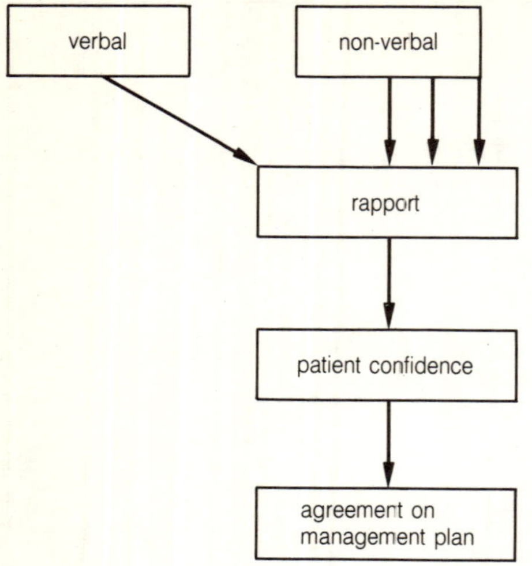


**Fig. A4.4** *Non-verbal influences are stronger than verbal.*

**The clinical method**

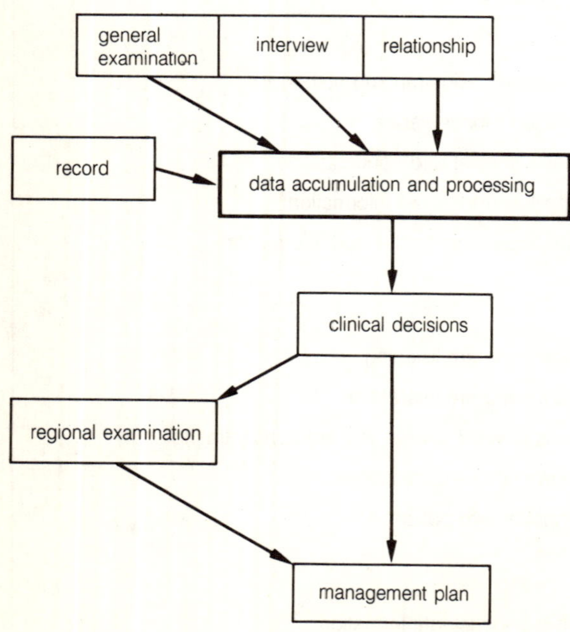


**Fig. A4.5**

**Social relations**

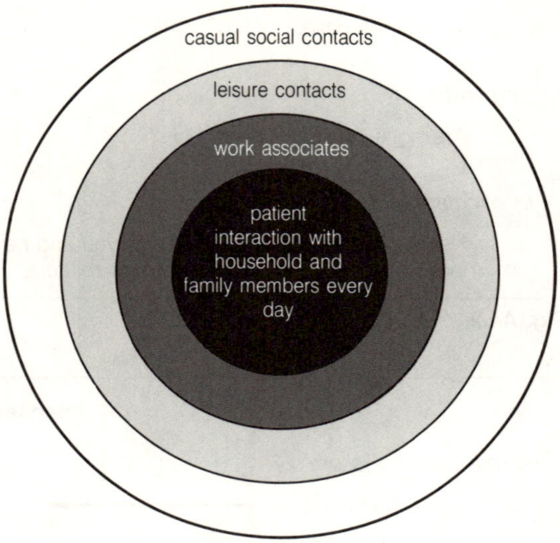

casual social contacts

leisure contacts

work associates

patient interaction with household and family members every day

**Intensity of social interaction**

| | |
|---|---|
| Most intense | 7 days per week with household members |
| Less intense | 5 days per week with work associates |
| Much less intense | 1–2 days per week with social associates |
| Least intense | with occasional social contacts |

**Fig. A4.6** *Every patient is the centre of a social circle.*

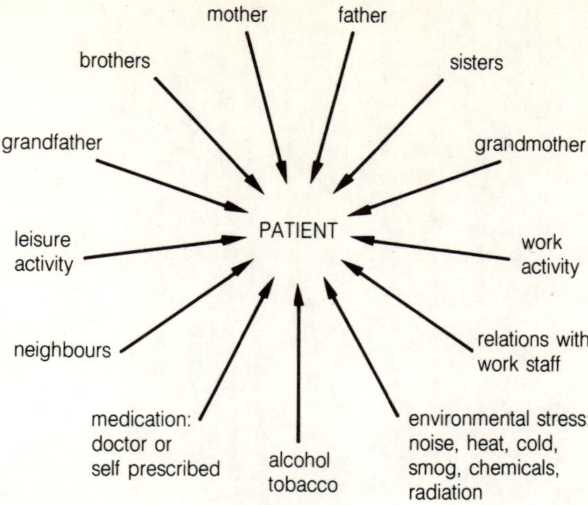


**Fig. A4.7** *Ask yourself if the symptoms have their origin in the patient or some other source.*

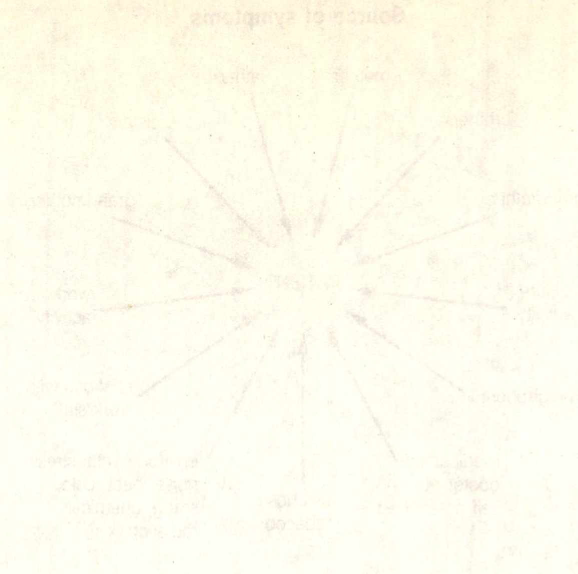

# Bibliography

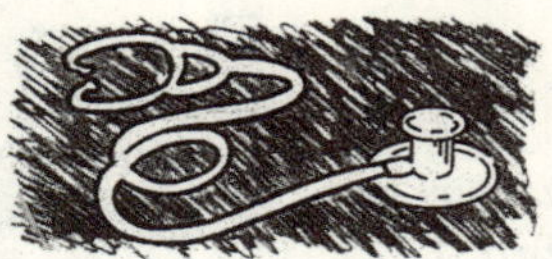

**Hodgkin, Keith**, *Towards Earlier Diagnosis in Primary Care*, 5th edn, Churchill Livingstone, Edinburgh, 1985.

This book is based on the author's meticulously kept records in hospital and general practice, and includes systematic consideration of specific diseases. It has much interesting material on the relative frequency of diseases in general practice as compared with hospital.

**Browne, Kevin & Freeling, Paul**, *The Doctor–Patient Relationship*, 2nd edn, Churchill Livingstone, Edinburgh, 1976.

This is a very readable, interesting book about the doctor–patient relationship at emotional level and certainly repays study.

**Argyle, Michael**, *The Psychology of Interpersonal Behaviour*, 4th edn, Penguin, Harmondsworth, 1983.

This book contains the results of detailed analysis of social behaviour over the last two decades. It is of value to anyone whose work involves dealing with people, such as interviewers, teachers, managers and doctors.

**Balint, Michael**, *The Doctor, His Patient and the Illness*, 2nd edn, Churchill Livingstone, Edinburgh, 1986.

This book demonstrated for the first time, in modern terms, the specific role which had always existed for GPs . . . to understand the whole of the patient's communication.

**Berne, Eric**, *Games People Play: The Psychology of Human Relationships*, Penguin, Harmondsworth, 1970.

This book is about transactional analysis. If you want to know what that is, read it; it's very readable, and important.

**Thouless, Robert H.**, *Straight and Crooked Thinking*, Pan Books, London, 1974.

This practical book by an eminent psychologist tells how to think clearly and avoid muddled reasoning. It exposes many dishonest tricks frequently used in argument.

**Fraser, Robin C.**, *Clinical Method: A general practice approach*, Butterworths, London, 1987.

This book is a series of essays on general practice by five contributors and contains much interesting material. It is based on general practice in the UK.

**Braunwald, E. et al. (eds)**, *Harrison's principles of Internal Medicine*, 11th edn, McGraw-Hill, New York, 1987.

**Nelson, Waldo E. et al. (eds)**, *Nelson Textbook of Pediatrics*, 13th edn, W.B. Saunders, London, 1987.

Both Nelson and Harrison are familiar to students and doctors as standard and very valuable reference texts. They continue to be valuable in general practice.

**Macleod, John (ed.)**, *Clinical Examination*, 3rd edn, Churchill Livingstone, Edinburgh, 1973.

This has become the standard students' clinical text in recent years and adopts a hospital perspective. It is useful as a reference text in general practice.

*ICHPPC-2-DEFINED (International Classification of Health Problems in Primary Care)*, 3rd edn, Oxford University Press, Oxford, 1983.

This sets out the classification of diseases developed by the International General Practitioners Organisation and has a potential as a research tool now that most classifications have agreed criteria. It provides the potential to determine optimum treatments of common diseases.